Comments on **Parkinson's a** ▮▮▮▮▮▮▮ *aders*

'In my opinion this book strikes a perfect balance between information and sympathy, without being too technical or too maudlin. I feel sure that this book will become a vade mecum for anyone associated with Parkinson's, whether it be the patient, carer, GP or therapist.

I feel sure that it will fill a very much needed gap in the market for educating and reassuring all those who are involved in any way with Parkinson's.'

Dr Lloyd A. Frost, Leeds

'I found the book easy to read and comprehensive. Patients and carers must take the information and demand or even, with the help of others, set about making it happen themselves, if they wish to get the best of what is available. A super DIY manual for patients and carers.'

Dr Bernard Dean, Kimbolton, Cambridgeshire

'I have learned a good deal about my own troubles which is a great help.'

Lois Buckley, Alresford, Hampshire

'A good attempt to answer the questions people with Parkinson's have – it will be especially useful for people who are newly diagnosed.'

Keith Levett, Bath

'I think the newly diagnosed person will find it most helpful and it will dispel any fears they may have had. I wish you every success with the publication of this most important book.'

Les Pickford, Hornchurch, Essex

GW00632190

Parkinson's at your fingertips

THE COMPREHENSIVE PARKINSON'S REFERENCE BOOK FOR THE YEAR 2000

Marie Oxtoby BSc(Soc), PhD
Social researcher; Chairman of the Parkinson's Disease Society's Welfare Advisory Panel and of the Bolton Branch; former Director of the Romford Neuro-care Project

Adrian Williams MD, FRCP
Professor of Clinical Neurology, Queen Elizabeth Hospital, Birmingham; member of the Parkinson's Disease Society's Medical Advisory Panel

CLASS PUBLISHING · LONDON

© Marie Oxtoby, Adrian Williams 1995
All rights reserved

The rights of Marie Oxtoby and Adrian Williams to be identified as the
authors of this work have been asserted by them in accordance with the
Copyright, Designs and Patents Act 1988

Printing history
First published 1995

The authors and publishers welcome feedback from the users of this book.
Please contact the publishers.
Class Publishing, 7 Melrose Terrace, London W6 7RL, UK
Telephone: 0171 371 2119
Fax: 0171 371 2878 [International +44171]

A CIP catalogue record for this book is available from the British Library

ISBN 1 872362 47 8

Designed by Wendy Bann

Edited and indexed by Susan Bosanko

Cartoons by Linda Moore

Line illustrations by David Woodroffe

Production by Landmark Production Consultants Ltd, Princes Risborough

Typesetting by DP Photosetting, Aylesbury, Bucks

Printed and bound in Great Britain by Clays Ltd, St Ives plc

Contents

Acknowledgements

All books are team efforts and this one is no exception. Although it is impossible to name everyone who has contributed to the preparation of this book, we would like to acknowledge our particular debt to the following people.

People with Parkinson's and others who provided a wide-ranging selection of questions. We are particularly grateful to all the people with Parkinson's and their families, from whom we have learned - and continue to learn - so much, and would like to dedicate this book to them.

Members of YAPP&RS for responding to requests for questions and their chairman Keith Levett for reading the manuscript.

Bridget McCall (Information Officer) at the Parkinson's Disease Society for prompt practical assistance in retrieving information, patient reading of drafts and redrafts, and unstinting moral support and encouragement.

Franklin MacDonald (Welfare and Benefits Adviser), Anne Mathon (Counsellor) and other staff members at the Parkinson's Disease Society for relevant questions and much specialist information and advice.

Jane Stewart (Nurse Specialist Project Coordinator) for specialist information on apomorphine and Parkinson's Nurse Specialists.

Doctors Lloyd A. Frost, Hardev Pall and Andrew Lees for reading the manuscript and making helpful comments and suggestions.

Linda Moore, our cartoonist, for being the only member of the team to meet her deadlines and for inspiring us with her perceptive and humorous cartoons.

Les and Lilla Pickford for agreeing to be photographed so that our commitment to reality could extend to the book's cover.

Foreword

by Professor C.D. Marsden DSc, FRCP, FRS

Professor of Clinical Neurology, The National Hospital, Queen Square,
London; Chairman, Head, University Department of Clinincal Neurology,
Institute of Neurology, London

The impact of being diagnosed as having Parkinson's is profound. That event is the beginning of a lifelong journey in which the individual, their family, their carers, their friends and their professional advisers face a multitude of questions and problems. *Parkinson's at your fingertips* provides sensible answers to all the questions that everyone concerned with this journey will ask. What is the illness, how is it treated with drugs and surgery, what is the role of physical therapies and complementary medicine, how will it influence attitudes and relationships, work and leisure, the impact on financial arrangements and long-term plans are dealt with in this outstanding book. The style is exactly what people need, namely the posing of questions that are commonly asked followed by sensible and practical answers. The authors have particular expertise and interest in Parkinson's: this shines through in the way in which the questions are answered. They are to be congratulated on producing a volume which will be invaluable to everyone concerned with Parkinson's.

CJ Marsden

Foreword

by Mary G. Baker

Director of Welfare Development, Parkinson's Disease Society
of the United Kingdom

Do any of us really appreciate how much we value the control we have over our lives? Perhaps not, until we feel we are losing it.

Being diagnosed with a chronic deteriorating illness like Parkinson's Disease can be devastating and many people feel they are losing control. Coping with the impact of the diagnosis, understanding and managing the condition, the medication and the inevitable changes and uncertainties with which they are faced will necessarily involve a great many questions, for which people need clear and honest answers.

Parkinson's at your fingertips provides the answers to so many questions concerning the medical, social and personal needs of people with Parkinson's and their families.

Francis Bacon said 'knowledge itself is power'. This book will help empower people living with Parkinson's Disease. It will give them the information they need, increase their knowledge and understanding, and enable them to retain control and make informed choices about their lives.

xiii

Introduction

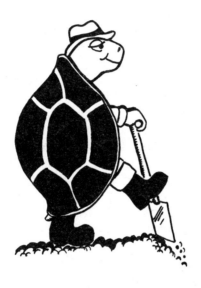

If you are someone who has Parkinson's, or if you have a relative or friend with Parkinson's, then this book is intended for you. Its starting point is the important questions which you and people like you ask every day. The questions are real questions we have been asked by real people and, in answering them clearly and honestly, we hope to improve your access to information and help so that you can get on with your life as normally as possible. We believe that if you are well informed and involved in decisions about your own care, your treatment will be more successful and you will feel more in control. We also hope that the information in this book will be of interest to the doctors, nurses, therapists and other professionals who work with people like you, and will help them to be more aware of the everyday implications of living with Parkinson's.

Parkinson's is an extremely complicated and variable condition and people can and do live with it for 20 years and more. Being diagnosed does not mean that someone's symptoms will get worse – in fact the reverse is more likely to be true. Although there is as yet no cure, there are some effective treatments and more are being developed. No two people are exactly alike either in their symptoms or in their response to treatment, so the questions and answers in this book cover a vast range of situations from the most mild to the most serious. It is impossible for anyone to suggest any one treatment or course of action which would be right for everyone, and we have not tried to do so. Instead we have tried to provide you with information about the various options that are available, and the organisations and people to whom you can turn for more detailed and more personal help and advice.

The medical condition with which we are concerned in this book is Parkinson's Disease. It is named after Dr James Parkinson, a remarkable and talented London doctor who, in 1817, first properly described its main features and outlined the course of the illness. However, you will notice that we refer throughout to Parkinson's rather than Parkinson's Disease. This is because we know from experience that many people are distressed by the word 'disease' and would find its constant repetition distracting and upsetting. Although the medical textbooks are unlikely to change, many voluntary organisations around the world now use this shortened name. It is certainly easier to say and this book will also be several pages shorter as a result of our decision!

Neurology, the branch of medicine involved with Parkinson's, uses many very technical terms to refer to the complex range of symptoms and side effects. We have used, and explained, those terms which are in most frequent use (there is also a glossary at the back of the book for easy reference) but otherwise we have tried to avoid technical language and jargon.

Drug names are also confusing – and subject to change. Most drugs have at least two names, the generic or true name and the trade (or brand) name given by the company which makes the drug. Usually we give both versions, using small first letters for the generic name and capital first letters for the trade name.

Parkinson's at your fingertips may strike some people as a rather odd title, as one of the symptoms of Parkinson's is that it can make fine movements of the fingers more difficult. The reason for the title is that the book belongs to a series of books about different conditions, all of which are intended to provide accessible and reader-friendly information (you will find details of other books in the series at the back of this book). We hope that we have succeeded in this aim! Evidence that people with Parkinson's can use their fingers very effectively is provided by our cartoonist, Linda Moore, a younger person with Parkinson's who works as a teacher and leads a very active life. We hope that you like her drawings as much as we do and that you will be encouraged by her constructive and sometimes humorous approach to Parkinson's. She chose the tortoise as her 'character' because slowness is an important feature of the condition but also because, as the fables remind us, tortoises always get there in the end!

How to use this book

The book is not intended to be read from cover to cover but to be used selectively to meet your own particular situation. It has a detailed list of contents and a comprehensive index so that you can quickly identify the parts which are relevant to you. For example, people who are newly diagnosed might want to find out more about the nature of Parkinson's (in Chapter 1), its main symptoms (in Chapter 2) and the treatment they have been given (in Chapter 3). They may also want to look at Chapters 4 and 5 which address questions of access to treatment and of attitudes and relationships. People still at work might want to concentrate on the appropriate section of Chapter 7, and may find some of the financial information in Chapter 11 useful. The carers of people with advanced Parkinson's will find helpful information about support for carers in Chapter 5, advice on benefits in Chapter 11, and discussion of options for care outside the home in Chapter 12.

Please remember that a book like this cannot provide exact and full answers to your individual problems. What it can do is to provide you with the information which will help you to obtain those answers from doctors, health professionals and workers in the voluntary and statutory services in your own area.

Not everyone will agree with the answers we give, but future editions of this book can only be improved if you let us know when you disagree and have found our advice to be unhelpful. We would also like to know if there are important questions we have not covered. Please write to us c/o Class Publishing, 7 Melrose Terrace, London W6 7RL, UK.

1
What is Parkinson's?

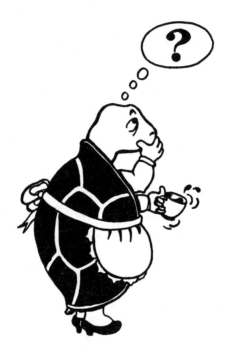

Introduction

This chapter tries to address some difficult questions about the nature of Parkinson's – difficult because we do not yet know all the answers. We have tried to be honest where this is the case and those interested in research developments can turn to Chapter 13 where the continuing search for answers is discussed further.

The cause - or causes - of Parkinson's

What goes wrong in Parkinson's?

In Parkinson's, a small part of the brain called the substantia nigra (see Figure 1) loses a lot of its nerve cells and so is unable to function normally. These nerve cells use a chemical known as dopamine to send messages to other parts of the brain and spinal cord which control coordination of movement.

The substantia nigra has been described as the gearbox of the brain. When it stops working properly it leads to tremors (shaking), over-rigidity of the muscles (stiffness), slowness and uncoordinated movement. These effects often show up as difficulties with arm and leg movements or, less often, as problems with speech. Remember, though, that they will not all affect every person with Parkinson's. They often start on one

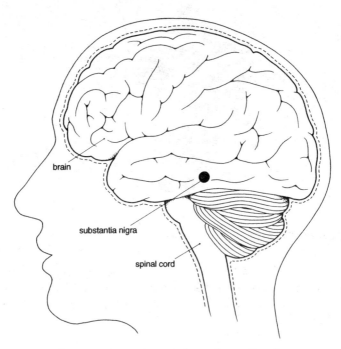

Figure 1: Location of the substantia nigra

side of the body and, although there is a general tendency for them to spread to the other side, they can sometimes remain on just the one side for many years.

What causes the brain to stop making dopamine?

Dopamine is made by the cells in the substantia nigra. Brain cells die all the time but, in Parkinson's, these particular cells die earlier than they should. We do not need all the cells to continue functioning normally and it is estimated that about 80% of the cells in the substantia nigra have to be lost before the symptoms of Parkinson's begin to show. After this point the remaining cells cannot produce enough dopamine to keep the body's motor system running smoothly. The question which research is still trying to answer is why these cells die. Possibilities include viruses, poisons in the environment and shortages of protective chemicals in the brain.

My father's Parkinson's appeared after he had had a bad accident at work and I have met other people with similar experiences, so can shocks cause Parkinson's?

We know that by the time the first symptoms of Parkinson's appear many of the cells in the substantia nigra have already died, so most researchers believe that the disease process has been happening unnoticed for several years. It is therefore unlikely that any shock (such as your father's accident) that happened immediately before the symptoms appeared has played much part in causing Parkinson's. However, a period of anxiety or depression could possibly bring on symptoms that otherwise would have appeared weeks or months later. This is easiest to understand in the case of tremor. We all have some tremor and if we are anxious, it will show. So if someone who is on the threshold of developing the tremor of Parkinson's gets upset, it is easy to see how this could become noticeable earlier.

I saw the word 'idiopathic' written before Parkinson's in my husband's medical notes. What does it mean?

The word 'idiopathic' simply means that the cause is not known. This is true for everyone with Parkinson's except those in whom it is caused by drugs or (very rarely these days) by encephalitis lethargica, so it is hardly necessary to use the term at all. Not knowing the cause of a disease is common and one could equally well use the term 'idiopathic' in front of diabetes or high blood pressure or many other illnesses. (Drug-induced Parkinson's is discussed in the answer to the next question, and there is more information about encephalitis lethargica later in this chapter.)

What is drug-induced Parkinson's?

As the name implies, this is a form of Parkinson's which is caused by taking certain drugs. The drugs involved are mainly those used for serious psychiatric problems, not the ones normally used to relieve anxiety or depression. It can also be caused by Stemetil (prochlorperazine) which is used to control dizziness, or Maxolon (metoclopramide) which is prescribed for nausea.

Drug-induced Parkinson's is not really Parkinson's although, by coincidence, some people with real Parkinson's may have taken some of these drugs for a short period. The difference is that in cases caused by these drugs the symptoms will wear off over a few weeks or months once the drug has been stopped.

There is another, rare, sense in which the phrase 'drug-induced Parkinson's' is used – a substance known as MPTP was taken by some American drug addicts in the early 1980s and caused symptoms almost identical to those seen in Parkinson's. There is more information about this in Chapter 13 on *Research and clinical trials*.

I hate the word 'disease' and felt very upset when given the diagnosis – it sounds like something infectious or catching. Is it?

Parkinson's is certainly not catching or infectious. At the moment, even a virus seems an unlikely cause for Parkinson's but, even if it were later shown to be a cause, it is inconceivable that it would be infectious to others.

'Disease' can sound a rather harsh word, especially as there are many more serious conditions which do not carry this label. The official title is unlikely to be changed although many people in Britain and around the world are now referring to the condition as Parkinson's or PD. Use the description which you find most acceptable and try to develop a positive attitude towards your condition. We know this can help, and we discuss it in more detail in Chapter 5 on *Attitudes and relationships*.

Who gets Parkinson's?

I know that they say Parkinson's is not hereditary but I have it and so do two of my cousins. How can the doctors be sure?

Researchers have looked carefully at people with Parkinson's and at their families and, in nearly all cases, there is no other member of the family with the condition. Certainly the illness is not hereditary in the usual sense of the term, in that neither the mother, father, brothers or sisters have had the illness. Someone who has been diagnosed need have no worries about their own children or siblings even if they are identical twins.

Having said that, if one looks in the wider family, for example cousins (as in your case), there is a slightly higher frequency of the illness than one would expect by chance. There are also very rare examples where one cannot doubt that Parkinson's is in the family. However, there are also cases in which everyone believes that there are several family members with Parkinson's but, on closer examination, it turns out that family members with a familial tremor (see Chapter 2 for more information about this) are being counted as if they had Parkinson's.

Could Parkinson's have a genetic component even though it is not hereditary?

Another way of putting this question might be: 'Could Parkinson's have something to do with a person's genes (the building blocks which determine a person's main characteristics), even though it is not handed down directly from parent to child?' This is an important question but it is impossible to give a simple answer.

Researchers went through a stage of thinking that the genetic component in Parkinson's was very small because it was very rare for both members of a set of twins to get the illness. However, this was true both of identical and non-identical twins. To really test whether or not there is a genetic component, one needs to see a difference between the two types of twins. As an example, if there was a strong genetic component, both members of sets of identical twins would get the illness much more frequently than non-identical twins. The numbers of twins found and tested was insufficient to come to a definite conclusion.

Most people now believe that, as with many other common conditions, Parkinson's is likely to have a genetic component which makes some individuals susceptible to something in the environment, perhaps a chemical or a virus. Intriguing though this is, it does not alter the fact that the risk of the children of people with Parkinson's also developing the condition is negligible.

Is Parkinson's more common in men than in women?

At each age Parkinson's is somewhat more common in men than in women. Some studies have suggested that men are twice as likely to get it. However, as women on the whole live longer than men, and as the disease gets commoner with age, there are just as many women as men alive with Parkinson's.

I read somewhere that Parkinson's is found all over the world. Is this true or is it more common in some countries or climates?

Yes, Parkinson's is found worldwide. We do not always know what the exact figures are, as good research counting the number of people with Parkinson's is not available from every country. From what we do know, it does appear that Parkinson's is less common in countries closer to the equator than it is in the UK. However, moving to such countries will not help people with Parkinson's.

My sister is 37 and has been having trouble with her walking for some time. We thought it was a trapped nerve but now the

doctor says it is Parkinson's. I can't believe it - surely Parkinson's is an old person's disease?

At 37 your sister is certainly young to get Parkinson's, but it is by no means unheard of at that age, and all neurologists will have seen people with Parkinson's in their thirties and even younger. The illness is certainly much more common in the elderly but can affect those in relative youth. It is estimated that one in seven of those diagnosed are under the age of 40.

You will find many references throughout this book to the special problems and needs of younger people with Parkinson's and to a self-help group, the YAPP&RS, which brings them together and offers valuable support and encouragement. You will also find more information about the YAPP&RS in Chapter 14.

Recently we visited an old friend who has been told she has Parkinson's. She keeps asking herself 'Why me?' and wondering if there is anything she could have done to cause it. We reassured her that it was not her fault. Did we do right?

You were quite right to reassure her. It is natural to want an explanation for an illness and common for some people, particularly if they are a bit depressed, to be tempted to blame themselves. Bad habits certainly do not cause Parkinson's! Although we cannot yet answer the 'Why me?' question, nobody believes that the cause or causes of Parkinson's will turn out to be something under the control of those who get it. If your friend continues to blame herself, it would be worth you and her doctor considering whether or not she is depressed.

I am 68 and have always looked after myself. I do not smoke or drink to excess but now I am having all kinds of difficulties and the doctors have diagnosed Parkinson's. Why me?

'Why me?' is the crucial question for researchers to answer. At the moment all we can say to you is that it was more likely to have happened to you at your current age of 68 rather than 20 years earlier. Alcohol does not appear to be involved to any extent and the question of smoking is uncertain (see the answer to the next question). You are too young to have been involved in the epidemics of sleeping sickness (encephalitis lethargica) that were around at the time of World War I and which caused a special kind of Parkinson's. There has recently been some evidence that the body's inherited ability to turn harmful chemicals into harmless substances may be somewhat reduced in people who get Parkinson's but this is an area for future research rather than an established fact at present.

Is is true that smoking cigarettes can protect people from Parkinson's?

Some, but not all, research surveys have suggested that people who get Parkinson's have on the whole smoked remarkably little. One difficulty of these surveys is that they are biased because some smokers who should really have been included in the survey have already died of other causes, such as cancer. It is also possible that, before symptoms become obvious, there is something that makes individuals who are destined to get Parkinson's just not enjoy smoking. It remains a possibility that smoking genuinely protects people from getting Parkinson's but it is more likely that there is another explanation. One day we will be able to protect people from getting Parkinson's but smoking (which causes so much death and disability) will not be a part of the answer!

Outlook

Is there a cure for Parkinson's?

No, there is no cure yet. Most medical success stories are due to prevention rather than cure and this is particularly likely in neurological conditions (conditions affecting the body's nervous system) such as Parkinson's which are linked to the loss of nerve cells. To prevent something happening, we need to understand its cause, so research into the cause or causes of Parkinson's has to continue (see Chapter 13 on *Research and clinical trials* for more information about this). Meanwhile, there are treatments available (they are discussed in Chapter 3) so the overall situation is more favourable then in many other neurological conditions. Another hopeful development is that a way of slowing down the already fairly slow progression of Parkinson's symptoms may become available.

I have a tremor in one hand. Will it spread? Should I learn to write with my other hand?

As with other aspects of Parkinson's, tremor is a slowly progressive problem and, in the end, symptoms are likely to worsen and spread to the other side of your body. Parkinson's is very variable, so some people who start with tremor in one hand go for many years before it spreads to the other side, whilst in other people this happens more quickly. In a lucky few it stays on the one side.

Because of this unpredictability, it is difficult for us to answer the second part of your question. The possible long-term advantages of learning to use your other hand have to be weighed against the certainty that using your non-dominant side will make writing and other activities more difficult now. You might also find such efforts stressful, which could have an effect on your tremor (there is a question about the effects of stress in Chapter 2).

My brother, aged 48, was told he had Parkinson's a year ago. How quickly does it progress and could he end up in a wheelchair?

Most people with Parkinson's respond either well or very well to treatment, particularly when, as in your brother's case, it comes on at a fairly early age. You are probably going to see an improvement with treatment (rather than a deterioration) for several years to come. However, underneath this improvement, the dopamine nerve cells are gradually dying and eventually his response to treatment will tend to be less good. This may not become a problem for some five to 10 years.

The permanent use of a wheelchair is not common in Parkinson's. Although we cannot say for sure that your brother will never need to use a wheelchair, he is likely to be a good 20 years off any likelihood of needing one. Remember too that a wheelchair can extend, rather than limit, people's horizons – we discuss the practical aspects of mobility in Chapter 10 on *Getting around on wheels*.

Will I die from Parkinson's?

Parkinson's by itself does not cause people to die. Life expectancy with good treatment is not much changed from normal life expectancy, and none of the drugs that are used for Parkinson's have any serious side effects that could cause death. However, in people who are seriously disabled (usually those who have had Parkinson's for many years), their general physical condition can make it somewhat more difficult for them to cope with other illnesses such as pneumonia and fractured bones.

2
Symptoms and diagnosis

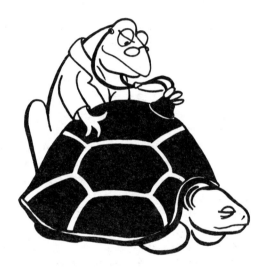

Introduction

No two people with Parkinson's are the same, and the initial symptoms in the first few years can vary markedly between different individuals. As time goes by, the differences in the way it affects people become even more noticeable, and certain symptoms and complications of treatment will simply **never** occur in many individuals. We also have to remember the effects of ageing – as people get older, some of the symptoms attributed to Parkinson's may really be caused by the ageing process itself, or by some other illness. This is particularly true of symptoms such as bladder problems, memory disorders, confusion, and aches and pains, where Parkinson's may be only one of several factors involved.

It is therefore very important that, as you read or dip into this chapter, you do not assume that you or your relatives will experience every symptom which is mentioned.

Problems of diagnosis

My Parkinson's was diagnosed four years ago but I was attending my doctor for two years before that. Is it difficult to diagnose?

The diagnosis of Parkinson's can be difficult and it is very common for people to realise, after the diagnosis has been made, that the symptoms have been there for longer than was first thought. These earlier symptoms could have led to your visits to the doctor, especially as some of them are rather vague and easily attributable to getting older, or to being a bit depressed, or they may have an arthritic flavour to them. The cause of a tremor can be difficult to diagnose as there is a common variety of tremor known as familial or essential tremor (see the next question for more information about this) which can be confused with Parkinson's.

As there is no laboratory test for Parkinson's, a doctor may not be able to be sure about the diagnosis until time passes and a change in the overall picture makes the Parkinson's more obvious or rules it out. Most doctors will not want to say it is Parkinson's until they are sure. This will usually be when at least two of the three main symptoms (tremor, slowness of move-ment and stiffness) are present.

What are the other medical conditions which sometimes get confused with Parkinson's?

There are several conditions that may need to be considered by your doctors.

- Essential tremor (otherwise known as familial or senile tremor) is a common cause of diagnostic confusion. Usually an essential tremor has been there, even if in a milder form, for many years and, in over half the cases, there is known to be a tremor in the family. By contrast, finding another member of the family with Parkinson's is rare. An essential tremor becomes worse with anxiety and rather better with small amounts of alcohol. Essential tremor is as its worst with the arms outstretched or when holding a cup of tea or writing, whereas the tremor of Parkinson's is usually most obvious when the arm is doing nothing and at rest (which is why it is sometimes described as a resting tremor). The tremor of Parkinson's is also quite often on one side. However, there are exceptions that make diagnosis difficult, particularly when the tremor appears to have come on recently but looks like an essential tremor. It is at this stage that the diagnostic skills of a specialist can be helpful but a totally confident diagnosis may still not be possible at the first consultation.

- A shuffling gait (looking rather like the one sometimes seen in Parkinson's) can occur in rather elderly people who are known to have had a stroke or high blood pressure. It is caused by hardening of the arteries rather than by Parkinson's. In such cases other symptoms that are often found in Parkinson's (such as tremor, stiffness and lack of coordination of movements other than walking) are usually absent.

- Some drugs can cause side effects that resemble Parkinson's. However, this form of Parkinson's will get better when the drugs are stopped, although the improvement may take many months. (There is a question about drug-induced Parkinson's in Chapter 1.)

- There are some rare conditions which are collectively known as the Parkinson's Plus syndromes, which begin by looking like Parkinson's but which then turn out to be untypical and which are harder to treat. The Parkinson's Disease Society is encouraging research into these syndromes and collecting together information for the people affected. Anyone who is told that they have one of these syndromes, such as Multiple

System Atrophy or Steele-Richardson Syndrome (they also have a number of alternative names, which are listed in the *Glossary*) should get in touch with the Information Officer at the Society (see Appendix 1 for the address and telephone number).

I know Parkinson's is something to do with the brain and I thought the doctor at the hospital would send me for a brain scan but she didn't. Why not?

The substantia nigra (the part of the brain affected in Parkinson's) is very small and cannot be seen on the type of brain scans that are available at the moment. One type of scan, the Computed Tomography (CT) scan, looks normal in someone with Parkinson's. Such scans are therefore only used when the doctor has a serious worry that it could be another condition such as a brain tumour, a blockage of the system that drains the fluid in the brain, or a stroke. These concerns are rare so, for most people, a brain scan is not necessary.

My friend has recently been told he has Parkinson's and he was sent up to a special clinic in London to have his tremor measured. What good will that do?

Your friend has probably been asked to go to the clinic as part of a research study to measure his tremor more accurately than a doctor can do in an ordinary clinic. Such careful measurements contribute to our understanding of Parkinson's and other neurological conditions, but they are not necessary for the diagnosis of Parkinson's. Your friend may, however, derive overall benefit from seeing doctors with a special interest in Parkinson's.

What should I do – my doctor says that I have Parkinson's but my friends don't believe it and really I don't either?

All doctors accept that their patients can be correct when they do not believe a diagnosis, particularly one for which there is no special test. The thing to do would be to go back to your GP and ask him or her how sure they are about the diagnosis. Parkinson's can usually only be diagnosed with reasonable certainty when two of the three main symptoms are present (see the next question for more information about them). If it is a problem of tremor with no other symptoms or physical signs, your GP may accept that the diagnosis cannot be substantiated with confidence. By the end of the discussion you may both have decided that it would be worthwhile to get the opinion of a specialist. If you have already seen a specialist and still do not believe or accept the diagnosis, you can ask for a second opinion under the NHS. If your GP and one or two specialists all agree that it is Parkinson's, you should probably accept that your friends might be wrong!

The main symptoms

An aunt in America has just written to say she has Parkinson's. I gather it is a complex condition and varies a lot between people, but what are the main symptoms?

You are quite right in saying that symptoms vary a lot between people. Symptoms relate to the three chief parts of Parkinson's – tremor or shaking, slowness and stiffness.

- Tremor or shaking, often mainly on one side, is a common early symptom. It is most obvious when the hand is at rest and may come and go. About half of the people with Parkinson's start off with a tremor and, although often obvious and embarrassing (because it happens when the hand is at rest), it is not as much of a problem as might be thought at first glance.
- Slowness of movement (bradykinesia) and lack of coordination is another sign of Parkinson's and creates more problems for people than the better-known tremor. Slowness can also be mainly on one side. Tasks take longer and require more concentration instead of being done automatically and without thinking. Difficulty with doing up buttons, brushing teeth or shaving are common ways in which the problem comes to light. Handwriting can be affected, becoming more

difficult, smaller and less legible. The technical name for the
type of smaller writing found in Parkinson's is micrographia.
- Stiffness (rigidity) of the muscles is the other major symptom.
  The arm may not swing normally whilst walking and this is a
  sign that the specialist often looks for carefully. A tendency to
  shuffle and to walk slowly is a common way for Parkinson's to
  appear, although falling is rarely a feature in the first stages.
  Facial expression often becomes less animated (the so-called
  'poker' or 'mask' face) and speech may become slower and
  more monotonous, though it usually remains compre-
  hensible.

**My father, who has come to live with us, has Parkinson's. I
think he is settling down but he does not look very happy and
hardly ever smiles. Is this the Parkinson's too?**

Almost certainly. Lack of facial expression is a feature of
Parkinson's (as mentioned in the previous answer) and is often
noticed first by relatives, particularly husbands or wives. While
it can be helpful to the specialist in making a diagnosis, it is a
distressing feature of the condition for the people themselves
and for their relatives and can lead to much misunderstanding.
We have discussed this important topic further in Chapter 5.

**I used to be proud of my handwriting and won prizes at
school. Now it is small and spidery. Can I blame Parkinson's
for this?**

Writing is often affected by Parkinson's. Characteristically it
does get smaller (micrographia), and so you can probably blame
your Parkinson's for the change in your handwriting.

There are other causes of handwriting problems although
they rarely have the effect of making the writing smaller. For
example, very trembly writing is usually caused by a form of
essential tremor rather than by Parkinson's. Difficulty with
writing which is unaccompanied by other problems is usually
caused by writer's cramp, which is a form of dystonia. (There is
more information about essential tremor in the previous section
of this chapter on *Problems of diagnosis* and more about
dystonia in the next section on *Other possible symptoms*.)

I love walking but now my feet do not always cooperate. How does Parkinson's interfere with walking?

Before we actually answer your question, we would like to stress how important it is for you to try and carry on walking, particularly as you like it so much. Keeping active, both mentally and physically, is a very important way of dealing with Parkinson's. You might find that having a companion with you on your walks or simply using a walking stick will give you extra confidence and there are further suggestions in Chapter 8 which could help.

Parkinson's can certainly affect walking in a number of ways through the combined effects of slowness and stiffness. As with most of the other features of Parkinson's, it varies enormously between individuals and usually responds well to treatment, especially in the early years.

The mildest way in which Parkinson's affects walking is through the loss of arm swing on either one or both sides, something which does not have any serious ill effects. In time the walking can slow down with a tendency to hunch the shoulders, and later it may develop into a shuffly, somewhat unsteady gait. At a more advanced stage, there may be particular difficulties with cornering, starting off and stopping, or going through doorways.

Sometimes when walking I stop suddenly and my feet seem to be stuck to the floor. I think it is called 'freezing'. What makes it happen?

You are quite right that this is known as freezing. Nobody understands quite why it happens. Sometimes it is triggered by being anxious or in an unfamiliar or crowded place. Approaching a doorway or negotiating confined spaces can create special problems, but at other times it can occur out of the blue. There are ways of trying to overcome it which we will discuss in Chapter 3 on *Treatment* and Chapter 8 on *Managing at home*.

I know that lack of balance and falling are fairly common among people with Parkinson's. Why should this be?

Loss of balance and falling are indeed features of Parkinson's, because the part of the brain which is affected by Parkinson's is one of the areas which is important for balance. However, such problems are very rare in the early years, nor do they happen to everybody, however long they have had the illness. Chapter 8 on **Managing at home** gives some ideas that may help you overcome the problem.

My husband's voice has become quite quiet but, more upsetting for me, is the loss of colour and expression. Is this a common feature of Parkinson's?

Some people with Parkinson's do get problems with their voices. It is rarely the first feature to be noticed and more often develops later when other parts of the body are more seriously affected. However, what you have noticed is not uncommon – that is that the voice becomes quiet and monotonous. The loss of colour and expression is upsetting for both the person with Parkinson's and for those who are close to them. There is often, but not always, a good reponse to drug treatment and speech therapy. Chapter 6 on **Communication** contains some suggestions that may help.

I take my tablets and get around fairly well but I get dreadfully tired and often cannot do the things I want. Why should this be?

Tiredness can be a feature of Parkinson's, particularly if your response to treatment has not been very good. The extra effort needed for actions which used to be spontaneous can be exhausting. It may be worth asking your GP or specialist whether you are taking as much medication as is desirable, or whether it would be worth taking more, at least for a trial period.

It is also possible that your tiredness is due to depression. Depression is an odd word which is often used differently by the man or woman in the street and by doctors. Sometimes people who would be diagnosed by doctors as depressed (and so considered for anti-depressant medication) do not think of themselves as depressed. Rather they complain of being tired all the time, or of the response to their treatment being less good than they expected. There is a question at the beginning of the next section about depression in Parkinson's.

Are the symptoms likely to be worse when I am feeling under stress?

Very much so. In Parkinson's, as in many aspects of life, stress is unhelpful: the more you are stressed, the worse your symptoms will appear to be. And just as anyone can tremble if they are very stressed, so stress is likely to exaggerate any tremor from your Parkinson's.

It is actually quite difficult for any of us to recognise when we are under stress. There may be occasions when your doctor thinks some of your symptoms are related to stress, even though you yourself do not feel particularly stressed at that time.

Many people who are under stress also sleep badly. Sleep is important in Parkinson's and, like most other people, you will probably feel better after a good rest. Keeping active and learning how to relax are important but if you have serious problems with sleeping, you should consult your doctor.

Other possible symptoms

How common is depression in people with Parkinson's?

Depression is common, and most people with Parkinson's will have some degree of it at one time or another. It can happen at any stage and indeed occasionally appears before the physical symptoms. For this reason it is generally believed to be part of the illness and not only a reaction to it – the chemical changes in the brain (which are connected with the Parkinson's) may lead to a biochemical form of depression. On the other hand any kind of illness, even a relatively mild one, can make people feel depressed and nearly everyone with Parkinson's will have their moments of low spirits. It is important to remember that depression is a fairly common illness in the general population, particularly among the elderly.

In part, any depression can be overcome with a combination

of a positive attitude and support and education about Parkinson's. In addition, some people with Parkinson's (just like many other people in the general population) may benefit from drug treatment for depression, and doctors may advise such treatment even for people who would not think of themselves as being depressed (we have discussed in the previous two questions how difficult it can be for any of us to recognise that we are either stressed or depressed).

Does Parkinson's affect the memory?

Sometimes memory difficulties can occur with Parkinson's. However, Parkinson's is often first diagnosed in people who are over the age of 55 – an age when many people have noticed that in any case their memory is not as good as it was! Fortunately, many compensate with the cunning of experience!

The other problem in answering this question is that once any of us start thinking about our memories, we can all find many things that we feel we ought to remember. The shock of developing any illness at all, particularly when it leads to some depression, would make anybody more introspective and so liable to make a mountain out of a molehill as far as memory is concerned. Memory problems can be a sign of depression and of anxiety.

Some of the rarer drugs given for Parkinson's, particularly anticholinergics such as Artane, can affect memory and for this reason they are not usually prescribed for elderly people (there is more information about anticholinergics in the section on *Other Parkinson's drugs* in Chapter 3). There are, however, some people with Parkinson's in whom serious and obvious memory problems raise concerns about more general mental deterioration.

I suffer badly from hair loss and my skin is constantly greasy. Could this be connected with my Parkinson's?

We don't know if you are a man or a woman, but in either case hair loss is not a particular feature of Parkinson's. In a man hair loss may be a natural effect of ageing (please see one of the authors!). In a woman it might be related to a general health problem, and we would suggest that you have a word with your GP.

A greasy skin can happen with Parkinson's but is not common and advice about careful skin care may help. Try washing with a mild, unperfumed soap and, if excessive dandruff is also a problem, you could try one of the special preparations, such as Selsun, available from the chemist. If the greasiness leads to irritation, you could ask your doctor to consider prescribing one of the lotions for dermatitis.

Can Parkinson's affect my eyes? I have got new glasses but still seem to have difficulty focusing sometimes.

Parkinson's does not directly affect the eye itself or the circuits for vision in the brain. However, the movements of the eyes can be affected to a slight degree in Parkinson's. This can lead to some problems turning the eyes inwards, which is necessary for reading. Any problems with focusing can usually be overcome by new glasses prescribed by a good optician who knows that you have Parkinson's.

Some Parkinson's medication (usually the anticholinergics) can cause poor focusing, as can some anti-depressants. If you have recently started on any of these drugs, it would be worth asking your GP whether they could have anything to do with your eye problems. As with many other problems, you should not automatically assume that your Parkinson's is the culprit.

If your visual problems are more serious than those we have discussed, and your optician or GP cannot explain them, you should ask to be referred to an eye specialist for an opinion.

I can cope with the Parkinson's but get a lot of discomfort from constipation which seems to have got worse since I was diagnosed. Could there be a connection?

Yes, there could be a connection. Constipation is a very common complaint among people with Parkinson's, although often (as in your case) there has been a tendency to it beforehand. We would have hoped that your treatment for Parkinson's might have improved things a little but that does not seem to be the case. It may be that you have been prescribed one of the Parkinson's drugs which can make constipation worse. These include the anticholinergics, so if you have been prescribed one of these it might be worth having a word with your doctor (there is more information about anticholinergics in the section on *Other Parkinson's drugs* in Chapter 3).

Eating a healthy diet is important for everyone with Parkinson's and can also help with constipation (see Chapter 9 on *Eating and diet*). Medication for your constipation is necessary and important if you are getting a lot of pain, and your doctor or your chemist can advise you about this. Try not to get too anxious about how often you open your bowels, though we do understand how this can happen when you have had painful bouts of constipation.

My husband suffers badly from cramp, especially at night. Could this be anything to do with his Parkinson's?

Ordinary muscle cramps can certainly be a painful problem. They may respond to treatments such as quinine (from your doctor) or to vigorous massage or simply to moving around.

However, there is a second type of leg cramp in which the foot turns inwards and for which the above treatments are unlikely to be as effective. It is also fairly common, but usually happens in the morning rather than at night. It is this type of cramp, known as dystonia, which is found most frequently in Parkinson's (although both types occur). If your husband's cramp is dystonia, then you will probably find that his foot gets stuck in one position.

So what is dystonia and is it related to Parkinson's?

Dystonia is an involuntary contraction of the muscles which causes the affected part of the body to go into a spasm. In the case of the leg, it is the foot that turns inwards. In the case of the hand and fingers, the wrist usually bends at an angle. It can also affect the neck (so that it twists) or the eyes (so that they go into spasm and cannot be opened easily). The dystonia seen most frequently in Parkinson's is in the foot; the next most common (although quite rare) affects the eyes. These dystonias do not appear to be caused by drugs and are a feature of the illness. We know this because very occasionally they are seen even before Parkinson's treatment has started.

Treatment for dystonia is not always easy. However, dystonia in Parkinson's can be a sign of not enough medication, so if you have this problem it would be worth talking to your doctor to see if you could try increasing your dose.

My mother who is 84 and has had Parkinson's for many years has begun to get very restless and has 'jumpy legs'. Is this likely to be part of the Parkinson's or is it something else?

Your mother's symptoms are likely to be part and parcel of her Parkinson's. Such movements are common in people who have had the condition for many years. Nobody fully understands them, but they are partly a side effect of the dopamine replacement therapy and partly the result of some progression of the condition. Early in the course of the illness, doctors try to prevent them by adjusting the medication but, later on, it may be impossible to avoid them without causing increased slowing or freezing.

These movements are known by a number of different names – 'involuntary movements' is the most straightforward and the one we have used in this book, but you may also hear them referred to as 'dyskinesias' or 'choreiform movements'. They can affect most of the body or just one part of it, and may affect different parts at different times. They can appear at certain times of the day, and when they occur is sometimes (although not always) linked to the timing of the last dose of dopamine replacement medicine (ie Madopar or Sinemet). We discuss the link between involuntary movements and treatment further in Chapter 3.

There are two other unlikely – but possible – causes for the symptoms you describe. The first is that they are common in drug-induced Parkinson's (there is more information about this condition in Chapter 1). The second is that there is another medical condition called 'restless leg syndrome'. Nobody understands what causes it and it also occurs in people who do not have Parkinson's, when it occasionally responds to a different type of medication called clonazepam.

My husband who has Parkinson's is 82 and has developed a new and distressing symptom. Every afternoon he starts getting very hot and feels an inner – not outer – burning. He becomes very distressed and his breathing is affected. It used to go on for a few hours and a rest in bed seemed to relieve him, but in the last few days he has taken longer to recover.

The symptoms your husband is getting are not well understood by doctors, but they are recognised as being a part of Parkinson's. They appear to be part of the Parkinson's itself, but they also appear to be a reaction to the drugs used to treat Parkinson's. However, stopping the drugs altogether (even when it is possible) rarely helps. Sometimes, but not always, this symptom occurs when people are getting involuntary movements.

We are sorry to have to say that there is very little that can be done to relieve this symptom. We can, however, reassure your husband that it is not a sign of his Parkinson's getting worse or of another illness. We hope that this reassurance is of some help and that it may relieve some of the understandable anxiety which you are both feeling.

My wife has had Parkinson's for 10 years and has recently lost a lot of weight. The doctor says that there is nothing else wrong but she cannot seem to put on any weight. Is this a common problem?

People with Parkinson's sometimes lose 10 or even 20 pounds in weight. Weight loss can occur at any stage and often happens over a fairly short period and then stabilises. It appears to be part of the Parkinson's and is hardly ever a separate cause for concern. This is even more likely to be the case if your wife has not lost her appetite. If, however, she has gone off her food, then it could be that she is suffering from depression and that her doctor should consider treatment for this.

You do not say if your wife is getting involuntary movements. These can be a cause of weight loss in Parkinson's, as all movement uses up the energy we take in from our food. It does not matter if the movement is involuntary or if we choose to take exercise, it all has the same effect.

Overall, then if your wife is eating a well-balanced diet (see Chapter 9 on *Eating and diet* for more information about this), if her own doctor is satisfied that there is no other cause for concern, and if her weight loss does not go on and on, we feel that it is best for you just to accept your wife's new weight and not make a thing of it. Forcing her to eat more can become self-defeating.

I have had Parkinson's for nine years and just recently have had some problems with swallowing. It is very embarrassing and distressing. What could be causing it?

Swallowing problems are not that common in the early years, but if you have had Parkinson's for nine years, then Parkinson's is the likely culprit. Nevertheless, as it is not common, doctors normally advise an examination by a throat specialist to make sure there is no other cause. It could, for example, be an easily treatable condition such as a piece of food or other foreign body stuck in the throat. However, if the specialist does not find anything – and they usually do not – then advice from a speech and language therapist can be very helpful as he or she can teach you some 'tricks' that may help.

As with other unpleasant experiences, once you have had this happen a few times, you may get into a vicious cycle of getting over-anxious about it. The therapist can help you feel more in control and so get back to eating more normally. It is extremely rare for swallowing problems in Parkinson's to cause danger from choking.

You will find information about how to get in touch with a speech and language therapist in Chapter 4 on *Access to treatment and services* and some more information on dealing with your problem in the section on *Eating and swallowing* in Chapter 9.

Is there a link between Parkinson's and Alzheimer's?

This is a straightforward question to which it is impossible to give a straightforward yes or no answer.

Alzheimer's is the commonest cause of dementia (sometimes called brain failure), in which the brain cells die more quickly than in normal ageing. The main symptoms are loss of memory and the loss of the ability to do quite simple everyday tasks. The cells affected in dementia are **NOT** the cells in the substantia nigra that are affected in Parkinson's.

Parkinson's and Alzheimer's are both more common in elderly people so, if you look at a group of elderly patients with Parkinson's, you will find a proportion who do have memory loss, confusion, and disorientation in time and space – a type of dementia. This would be a higher number than if you looked at another group of elderly people who did not have Parkinson's. There are probably several reasons for this, including the drugs used to treat Parkinson's. Nearly all the drugs used can cause confusion in some people although the anticholinergic drugs are especially suspect (there is more information about anticholinergics in the section on *Other Parkinson's drugs* in Chapter 3). When Parkinson's drugs are to blame, people usually get visions or other sorts of hallucinations, and if these are distressing, it may be necessary to change or withdraw the medication. Very rarely, Parkinson's can affect other parts of the brain and lead to other kinds of dementia.

Is it true that 'pure' Parkinson's is rare and that most people with Parkinson's also have other conditions as well?

Yes, this is an inevitable consequence of the fact that Parkinson's mainly affects people over 60. The older you are when you get Parkinson's, the more likely you are to already have other medical conditions as well. After your diagnosis, you will not be immune from getting other illnesses, so every symptom you have should not be blamed on your Parkinson's. It can be quite difficult to sort out the overlapping symptoms but anything new should be discussed with your doctor and properly investigated. Problems with eyesight, bladder, swallowing, or confusion can all be caused by Parkinson's, but they can also be caused by other things for which there are specific, effective treatments.

3
Treatment

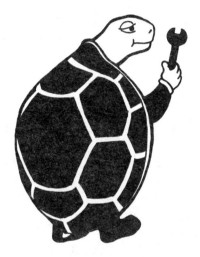

Introduction

This chapter will deal with a variety of treatments, concentrating on the standard types (drug treatment and the physical therapies) but also touching on the rarer surgical interventions and on the wide range of complementary therapies.

Parkinson's is one of the few neurological conditions for which specific drug treatments are available and, although they do not cure the condition or halt its underlying progression, they can make a huge difference to the symptoms and greatly improve people's quality of life. It is important to remember the point we made in our introduction to this book (and have repeated several times since!) – that Parkinson's varies greatly from one person to another. It is impossible for anyone to suggest any one treatment which would be right for everyone. Two people whose symptoms look similar and who have been diagnosed for approximately the same length of time may need different drugs and different doses.

The same is true for the physical therapies. We can give an overview, but there will be individuals who are not helped by the therapies that help most people, and others who seem to respond to treatments which are generally considered to have little value. The important thing is to work together with your specialist, GP and other members of the health team to discover what works for you or your relative.

L-dopa, Sinemet and Madopar

What is the most frequently used drug treatment for Parkinson's?

The most frequently used drugs are Sinemet and Madopar. Both of these drugs contain L-dopa, a compound one step removed from dopamine, the chemical messenger which is in short supply in Parkinson's (you will find more information about dopamine in Chapter 1). Once the L-dopa reaches the brain it is changed into dopamine, so making up for the shortage. Sinemet and Madopar are therefore a form of replacement therapy – like insulin in the treatment of diabetes. The various versions of Sinemet and Madopar, together with some other rarely used forms of L-dopa, are listed in Figure 2 (which gives both their trade and generic names, and the forms and sizes in which they are available).

Although these two drugs are the most used, not everyone with Parkinson's takes them. There are several other drugs available which may be more appropriate for some individuals at certain stages, and we discuss these later in this chapter.

TRADE NAME	GENERIC NAME	TABLETS OR CAPSULES	SIZES AVAILABLE
Sinemet	co-careldopa	Tablets	110 mg, 125 mg, 275 mg
Sinemet LS	co-careldopa LS	Tablets	62.5 mg
Sinemet CR	co-careldopa CR	Tablets	125 mg, 250 mg
Madopar	co-beneldopa	Capsules	62.5 mg, 125 mg, 250 mg
Madopar dispersible	co-beneldopa	Tablets	62.5 mg, 125 mg
Madopar CR	co-beneldopa CR	Capsules	125 mg
Brocadopa	L-dopa	Capsules	125 mg, 250 mg, 500 mg
Laradopa	L-dopa	Tablets	500 mg

Figure 2: Drugs containing L-dopa

Some comments on the drugs listed in the table.

- LS means low start: these versions of the drugs contain a small amount of L-dopa and are often used in the early stages of treatment.
- CR means controlled release, and we discuss these versions of the drugs later in this section.
- Co-careldopa is a shorthand way of saying 'L-dopa with carbidopa', and co-beneldopa 'L-dopa with benserazide'. Carbidopa and benserazide are examples of dopa-decarboxylase inhibitors, which are again discussed later in this section.
- Brocadopa and Laradopa are hardly used nowadays, so do not be surprised if you have not heard of them before.

What is the difference between Sinemet and Madopar?

Both Sinemet and Madopar contain two separate kinds of drug. The first, as explained in the previous answer, is L-dopa.

The second drug is there to prevent the side effects caused by taking L-dopa on its own. To make use of the L-dopa, the body has to change it into dopamine, and it can do this because it also makes another substance called dopa-decarboxylase. When L-dopa was first discovered, it was given on its own but, because it was being changed in the blood stream before reaching the brain, there were unpleasant side effects, particularly vomiting and low blood pressure. The discovery of other compounds which would stop the dopa-decarboxylase working until the blood carrying the L-dopa reached the brain was an important breakthrough in preventing these side effects. For obvious reasons, these compounds are called dopa-decarboxylase inhibitors.

Sinemet and Madopar use different dopa-decarboxylase inhibitors: the inhibitor in Sinemet is called carbidopa, and the one in Madopar is called benzerazide. However, the important thing to understand is that as far as the brain is concerned both drugs produce the same amount of dopamine. In spite of this, among the few people who have tried both Sinemet and Madopar, there are some who have a preference for one or the other. However, there is rarely any need to swop from one to the other.

What advantages do the new 'controlled release' versions of Madopar and Sinemet offer?

We first ought to explain the difference between the 'ordinary' versions of these drugs and the controlled release versions. When you swallow the ordinary version of Sinemet or Madopar, the amount of the drug in your blood stream rises in about half an hour, and then drops over the next hour or so. The controlled release versions simply keep the amount of the drug in your blood stream at a steadier level.

The new versions were developed when it was noticed that, after a few years of satisfactory treatment, people were getting less reliable benefits from their medication. Efforts were made to develop forms of Sinemet and Madopar that remained at a more steady level in the blood stream, and the result was the controlled release versions of these drugs. They do succeed in keeping the drug in the blood stream for longer but the effect on fluctuating symptoms has been somewhat disappointing. Many people still need the 'kick start' of the ordinary forms where, although the drug goes up and down in the blood stream faster, it goes up higher than with the controlled release drugs. Some people will, however, get a more even response to their doses of medication if they take the controlled release versions, although most will need to take a mixture of controlled release and ordinary Madopar or Sinemet.

Some people who notice troublesome symptoms at night will find that these controlled release drugs can be helpful as they have a longer lasting effect. They are therefore most often used for the last dose of the day. Some specialists give them right from the beginning of treatment, when they work just as well as the ordinary versions.

Will I feel better straight away when I start taking Madopar?

The L-dopa group of drugs such as Madopar or Sinemet often work fairly quickly. Many people, but by no means everyone, will feel some benefit within a few hours or days. However, even if you do not get an immediate effect, you are likely to notice some improvement over a week or two. If by chance you still don't feel much better then, you need to review the situation with your doctor. Sometimes your doctor will want to build up the dose slowly over several months.

What kinds of side effects do you get with Sinemet and Madopar?

Because these drugs put a natural compound back into the body, side effects at the beginning of treatment are rare. In the 1960s, when L-dopa was given alone, vomiting and low blood pressure (with consequent fainting) were common.

However, as explained earlier in this chapter, the addition of the dopa-decarboxylase inhibitors in Sinemet and Madopar has largely resolved these problems. Some people still get slight nausea or a little flushing right at the beginning of treatment. A few people are very sensitive to the drugs and decide to discontinue them. However, if you are one of these people, do not exclude the possibility of trying an L-dopa preparation a second time. Sometimes people in this situation do very well on their second attempt by starting with a lower than normal dose and building it up slowly.

Too much Sinemet or Madopar can cause involuntary movements (there is more information about involuntary movements in Chapter 2 and in the section on *Long-term problems* later in this chapter). Everything possible should be done to avoid this in the early years of treatment, but later on it may be necessary to put up with some involuntary movements in order to remain mobile. Such movements are not a simple side effect of the drugs but rather a mixture of the effects of the disease and of the medication. The same is true for the phenomena known as 'wearing off' and the 'on/off' syndrome (discussed in the section on *Long-term problems* later in this chapter).

How do I know if the side effects are normal or not?

When the doctor first prescribes your drugs, he or she will probably explain what effects you may experience as your body adjusts to the medication. You may also have access to a short and straightforward booklet called *The Drug Treatment of Parkinson's Disease* (see Appendix 2 for details) which is published by the Parkinson's Disease Society. If you are in any doubt about what may happen, have a word with your doctor or specialist. With this, as with any other questions for your doctor, it can be a good idea to make a list of the points you wish to make so that you don't forget to raise them at your next appointment.

All drugs can have some side effects and these have to be balanced against the advantages in each individual case. As explained in the answer to the previous question, it is unusual for Sinemet and Madopar to cause serious side effects. If you get involuntary movements, especially in the early stages of treatment, you should consult your doctor as your dose of medication may need to be reduced.

Dopamine agonists (including apomorphine)

My doctor says there are some other drugs called dopamine agonists which can help. How do they work?

Dopamine agonists (sometimes called dopa-agonists) work in a different way from the replacement drugs like Sinemet and Madopar. They do not provide extra dopamine: instead they stimulate the parts of the brain where the dopamine works ('agonist' is a term used for drugs which have a positive stimulating effect on particular cells in the body).

Figure 3 lists the dopamine agonists that are currently available in tablet or capsule form. Bromocriptine (Parlodel) has been around for many years; the others have been developed more recently. Apomorphine (discussed later in this section) is also a dopamine agonist but is currently only available as an injection.

TRADE NAME	GENERIC NAME	SIZES AVAILABLE
Parlodel	bromocriptine	1 mg, 2.5 mg, 5 mg, 10 mg
Revanil	lysuride	0.2 mg
Celance	pergolide	0.05 mg, 0.25 mg, 1 mg

Figure 3: Table of dopamine agonists available as tablets or capsules

What are the main advantages and disadvantages of dopamine agonists?

There are two main advantages. Firstly, because these drugs remain in the blood stream and in the brain for longer than Madopar and Sinemet, they can be used for people who are having a fluctuating or unpredictable response to those medicines.

Secondly, dopamine agonists do not cause involuntary movements (there is more information about involuntary movements in Chapter 2 and in the section on *Long-term problems* later in this chapter) particularly in people who have never been on any form of L-dopa. Because of this advantage, trials are being carried out and some doctors are already preferring to prescribe a mixture of an L-dopa drug and a dopamine agonist to newly diagnosed people. By doing this they hope to manage with lower doses of the L-dopa drug and therefore to reduce the risk of later problems such as involuntary movements and fluctuating responses to medication.

The disadvantages of the tablet/capsule forms of dopamine agonists such as bromocriptine (Parlodel), pergolide (Celance) and lysuride (Revanil) are that most people find them less effective in removing their symptoms than Madopar or Sinemet; that they frequently cause side effects so have to be introduced very slowly; and that they may make the drug regimes of elderly patients with other illnesses too complicated.

Because of this complex mix of advantages and disadvantages, dopamine agonists are rarely used on their own. Many people who try them will finish up on a combination of a dopamine agonist and a reduced dose of Madopar or Sinemet.

Are the newer dopamine agonists like Revanil and Celance less likely to cause side effects?

We cannot give a direct answer to this question as a trial that directly compares the three main dopamine agonists has never been done. However, there is little evidence that any one dopamine agonist has any advantage over the others – they all appear to work equally well and to have the same side effects.

Which kinds of people can benefit from apomorphine?

The people who seem to benefit most are those who have bad 'off' periods but who are reasonably well when 'on'. It does not help everyone, but it is now often tried with people who have 'off' periods of half an hour or more and who have not improved after adjustments to their ordinary medication. As apomorphine (Britaject) currently has to be given by injection, the person with Parkinson's and their carer have to be able to cope with this and to learn how to do it. This sometimes involves staying in hospital for a few days, although an increasing number of potential users are now being assessed and trained on a day care or domiciliary (home) care basis.

What are the main advantages of apomorphine?

The main advantage of apomorphine is that it can act as a 'rescue treatment' when tablets or capsules fail to take effect. For people who are assessed as suitable, it will work within 10 to 15 minutes – much more quickly than tablets or capsules.

Because of this predictable response, it can sometimes help people with Parkinson's to go on working for longer than would otherwise be possible.

Does apomorphine have disadvantages too?

Yes. Its main disadvantage is that at the moment it can only be given by injection (other methods of delivery have been tried but have so far proved ineffective). This means that both the person with Parkinson's and their main carer need to be willing and able to give the injections. The technique and the confidence to use it can be taught (as we explain later in this section), but there are people who feel unable to face the prospect of having or giving regular injections. It is important to involve the main carer (who may be a partner or a close friend or relative) because there may be times when the person with Parkinson's is too rigid or immobile to give the injection.

Apomorphine also causes nausea and vomiting but this problem has been largely overcome by giving another drug called domperidone (Motilium) beforehand. Some people can even manage without the domperidone after a few months. Domperidone is a safe drug and, although it makes the drug regime a little more complicated, this is not really a disadvantage.

Another disadvantage is that the site of the injections can become rather sore and irritated, especially when a syringe driver is used. This problem can be reduced by diluting the apomorphine with an equal amount of saline (a sterile salt solution).

Is apomorphine addictive?

No.

I have been told that I may need to use a syringe driver for my apomorphine injections. What is a syringe driver?

A syringe driver (shown in Figure 4 overleaf) is a small, battery driven pump which can deliver a continuous dose of medication through a needle which is inserted under your skin (subcutaneously) in your lower abdomen (ie the area below your navel).

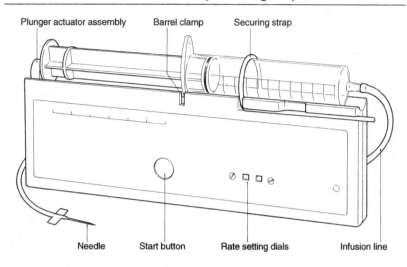

Plunger actuator assembly Barrel clamp Securing strap

Needle Start button Rate setting dials Infusion line

Figure 4: Syringe driver

The medication - apomorphine in Parkinson's - is then absorbed into your blood stream and goes from there to your brain. The dose can be adjusted to suit you, and the pump itself is carried in your pocket or in a small pouch. You need to change the position of the needle each day to reduce the risk of your skin getting sore. A small number of people use their syringe drivers continuously day and night. If this is essential, the needle site must be changed every 12 hours.

Only a minority of the people who are prescribed apomorphine need to use a syringe driver - mainly the people who have found that they need more than 10 injections a day. Changing over to a syringe driver can greatly improve the quality of their lives.

What are the alternatives to a syringe driver and how do they work?

There are two alternatives available at the moment. The first is a syringe of the type that people with diabetes use to give themselves their insulin. Most people who use apomorphine begin with this and many find it quite simple and easy to use.

The syringe can be carried in a toothbrush container and fits easily into pockets and handbags.

The disadvantage of a syringe is that it can only hold one dose. For this and other individually varied reasons, some people prefer to use a Hypoguard Penject, a special type of multi-dose syringe. As you can see from Figure 5, a Penject looks rather like a pen – hence the name. Some people with diabetes use similar devices (which they call insulin pens) to give themselves their insulin. The disadvantage of a Penject is that it can be rather fiddly to load, which may create problems for people with difficulties arising from tremor, stiffness or involuntary movements.

Both syringes and Penjects deposit the apomorphine (Britaject) just under your skin, and have the advantage of not irritating it as much as a syringe driver. They do not, of course, give you continuous medication, but you can repeat your apomorphine injection several times a day as necessary.

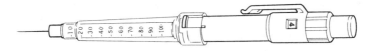

Figure 5: Penject

I have a severe tremor and live alone so measuring the correct dose of apomorphine would be difficult. Is there any solution to this problem?

If you are found to be suitable for treatment with apomorphine (Britaject), you will be trained in its use by your specialist hospital team or Parkinson's Nurse Specialist. They will show you how to prepare your Penject or syringes in advance – perhaps a whole day's supply at a time – which you can then store in the fridge until needed. This means that you can choose the time of day when you are at your best to measure the doses. If there are no times when you would feel able to manage this task, you could perhaps ask a friend or relative to help or, failing that, a community nurse could be asked to prepare them for you.

Can syringe drivers, syringes and Penjects be prescribed on the National Health Service?

There is little problem with prescribing the syringes as they are also widely used for diabetes. Penjects cannot be ordered on an ordinary prescription form: anyone who has any problems in obtaining them should contact the ward or clinic where they were assessed and trained and ask for further advice.

Syringe drivers are quite expensive and there are sometimes local problems in obtaining them. These problems are usually not insurmountable, although a certain amount of initiative may be required by you yourself, your doctor or nurse, or your local Parkinson's Disease Society branch. The fine infusion lines used with syringe drivers have to be obtained through the District Nursing Service.

Are there some special centres which provide training and support to apomorphine users?

In several areas of the country there are now neurologists or geriatricians (doctors who care for the elderly) with a particular interest in Parkinson's and it is likely that there will be some kind of special service for people who need apomorphine from the main hospitals or clinics where these specialists work.

In addition, some of these clinics and some GP group practices now have a Parkinson's Nurse Specialist (there is more about these nurses in the section on *Medical treatment and related services* in Chapter 4). One of her roles is helping and supporting people who are trying apomorphine. The Parkinson's Disease Society will know what is going on in your area, so contact them (address in Appendix 1) if you need more information.

Are there any new developments in the pipeline which will make apomorphine easier to use?

Yes. A special pen-type injection system which is pre-loaded with apomorphine (Britaject) is being developed and should be available shortly. People with diabetes already have access to these types of devices and they will be particularly helpful to people with Parkinson's who currently have difficulty preparing and using syringes and Penjects.

Many people hope that a different method of delivering apomorphine (ie other than by injection) will be found. Research is continuing in several medical centres around the world into oral (by mouth) and nasal delivery of apomorphine. However, it seems unlikely at the moment that such systems will offer the major advantage of injected apomorphine, which is its rapid action.

Other Parkinson's drugs

What other kinds of drugs are used in the treatment of Parkinson's?

So far we have discussed the drugs which contain L-dopa and the dopamine agonists. There is another, older, group of drugs called anticholinergics which work by reducing the amount of another chemical messenger, acetylcholine, thereby slightly increasing the amount of dopamine activity. There are a large number of these anticholinergic drugs of which the most commonly used are listed in Figure 6.

TRADE NAME	GENERIC NAME
Artane	benzhexol
Cogentin	benztropine
Akineton	biperiden
Disipal	orphenadrine
Kemadrin	procyclidine

Figure 6: Table of the most commonly used anticholinergic drugs

Although individuals may find one type or brand more suitable than another, in general no one stands out as better than the others. They are not used now nearly as much as they were before the discovery of L-dopa, and they tend to be avoided for elderly people as they can cause side effects such as confusion, dry mouth and difficulty in passing urine. Sometimes they are used alone in the early years before an L-dopa preparation becomes necessary, but they are more frequently used as an addition to L-dopa therapy. Anticholinergics can be useful to offset tremor or slowness of movement and can also be helpful when drooling (excessive salivation) is a problem.

It is not a good idea to stop anticholinergic drugs suddenly as this can lead to serious episodes of 'freezing' in which the person stops – as though rooted to the floor – and finds it difficult to get going again.

A neighbour who also has Parkinson's has been put on selegiline and says everyone with Parkinson's should have it. Is this correct?

This is another question which cannot be answered simply or completely. Selegiline (Eldepryl) was originally introduced as a drug which increases, to a small extent, the dopamine levels in the brain by blocking (stopping) the action of another naturally-occurring chemical (monoamine oxidase B or MAO B) which causes the breakdown of dopamine. By preserving the dopamine, selegiline can therefore cause a small improvement in symptoms and a slight ironing out of fluctuations in some people with Parkinson's. So although selegiline is nothing like as powerful as the L-dopa preparations or the dopamine agonists, it can be a good drug to use for newly diagnosed people with mild symptoms.

There is, however, another more complicated and controversial side to your question. In preventing the breakdown of dopamine, selegilene may also be reducing the amounts of a potentially damaging family of compounds known as 'oxygen free radicals' which could be involved in killing off the dopamine producing brain cells. If this theory could be proved, then selegilene would be the first drug actually to slow down the progression of Parkinson's. A big trial was therefore done in North America to see if newly diagnosed people who were given selegiline did better than newly diagnosed people who were given a placebo. The results were clearcut in that, after a year or two, the people who had been given selegilene were much less likely to have reached a stage where they felt in need of L-dopa treatment. How much of this was due to treating their symptoms and how much was due to actually slowing down the progression of their Parkinson's remains uncertain, although most researchers are now doubtful about the 'slowing-down' effect. Some authorities think that all people with recently diagnosed Parkinson's should be given selegilene, while others think that we should wait for more definite research results.

Anyone taking selegiline (Eldepryl) and later needing treatment for depression should ask their doctor to ensure that they are given an anti-depressant which is suitable for use with MAOIs (the group of drugs to which selegiline belongs).

General questions about drug treatment

My friend, who has had Parkinson's for the same length of time as me, takes twice as many tablets as I do. Can this be right?

People with apparently similar types of Parkinson's can often need quite different doses. The dose required for any particular person has little to do with the severity of the symptoms or with the length of time since diagnosis. In other words, it is not good or bad to be on more or less drugs. The doses which are right for you and for your friend are the ones which give you the most benefit with the fewest side effects.

I was brought up to avoid taking tablets and often read of the damage they do. Now I have been diagnosed as having Parkinson's and have been told that I will have to take tablets for the rest of my life. Can I refuse?

You are, of course, free to decide not to take Parkinson's – or any other – drugs and you should always be involved in decisions about your health care. Before attempting a fuller answer to your question, we should acknowledge that there are quite a few people who feel as you do. Medicines are such a big part of health care today that it is easy for health workers to take them for granted and to underestimate the fears and feelings of people like yourself.

There are several important points to make. First you should explain to your doctor how you feel and ask him or her to set out for you the likely consequences of taking or not taking the medication. There is certainly no hurry to start medication in most people and, as you will see from the previous answer, there is some controversy about the point at which drugs should be started and which drugs should be used in early, mildly affected people. No doctor is therefore going to mind if you want to wait. Alternatively you could compromise and try just selegiline (Eldepryl) which has a mild but definite effect on the symptoms.

Secondly, it is worth remembering that drugs containing L-dopa are a form of replacement therapy (putting back a natural compound) and they work reasonably well for most people. You might do yourself a disservice and reduce your quality of life if you wait too long.

Lastly, only you can know when the discomfort caused by your Parkinson's outweighs the discomfort you feel at being on permanent medication. Do not be afraid to return to your doctor if you decide to say no now but later want to change your mind.

Should I stop taking the tablets if they make me feel unwell?

We will assume that you have been given an idea of what to expect in the early days of trying a new tablet. If you feel more unwell than you expected, for example if you feel very sick or faint, go back to your doctor as soon as possible and ask if you can stop taking those particular tablets. Your doctor may try you on a different sort of drug instead, or may suggest that you try the same drugs again but at a lower dosage. Some people do very well on their second attempt by starting with a lower than normal dose and building it up slowly.

Once you have settled on the tablets, particularly when they have proved helpful, it is usually unwise to change them suddenly. If you feel very unwell after a period of stable and successful treatment, the chances are that something other than the drugs is causing your new symptoms. Go to see your doctor so that you can explore what is causing the problem.

Can I adjust the tablets myself to suit my activities or how I am feeling?

When you have a good knowlege of your Parkinson's and know the difference between being underdosed and overdosed, many doctors will encourage you to experiment a little yourself with the precise dosage and timing of your tablets. Your doctor may, for example, be able to tell you that your total daily dose of Madopar or Sinemet should be roughly so many tablets and encourage you to experiment a little while keeping within this daily total. How you split them up during the day and how you take them in relationship to meals can be varied until, by a little trial and error, you find out what suits you best.

How important is the timing of medication in Parkinson's?

The timing is not too critical in the early years but, as time goes on, it becomes extremely important for many people with Parkinson's. This is because they can experience great discomfort and immobility (see the next section on *Long-term problems* for further discussion of these problems) and so need access to their medication at very precise times. This means that they have to plan their lives and activities very carefully – a loss of spontaneity which some people find very frustrating.

Problems with getting medication at the right times are especially acute when people with Parkinson's are admitted to hospital, especially when they are on non-neurological wards. The anxiety and distress caused by poor timing of their medication can add considerably to the normal stress experienced by people in hospital. Efforts are being made to increase understanding of these problems among medical and nursing staff through seminars and through publications such as the Parkinson's Disease Society's *Information Pack for Nurses* (see Appendix 2 for details), but we still hear accounts of bad experiences. We discuss ways in which people going into hospital can minimise these problems in Chapter 12.

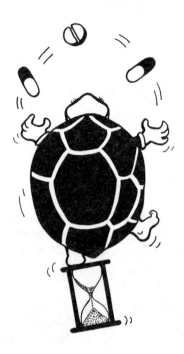

Is it all right to take other kinds of medicines at the same time as those for Parkinson's?

People with Parkinson's often have other conditions for which they need medication. Reassuringly, the drugs for Parkinson's are not upset by other kinds of medication. It is particularly important to stress that, if people with Parkinson's become depressed, there is no reason for them to avoid normal anti-depressant drugs if their doctors think that these will be helpful. You can also take painkillers and sleeping pills.

There are however a number of drugs (listed in Figure 7) which should almost always be avoided by people with Parkinson's. This is because they tend to bring on Parkinson's-like symptoms. The list includes some of the anti-depressant drugs, but there are many alternative ones available.

A word of caution is necessary here. We cannot guarantee that the list of drugs given in Figure 7 is exhaustive, as new drugs are being developed all the time. If you are offered a new drug by your doctor (or any drug which you have not had before, for that matter), it is always worth asking whether it is suitable for someone with Parkinson's.

TRADE NAME	GENERIC NAME	USUALLY USED FOR
Stemetil	prochlorperazine	Dizziness
Maxolon	metoclopramide	Vomiting
Motival ⎤ Motipress ⎦	fluphenazine and nortriptyline	
Parstelin	tranylcypromine and trifluoperazine ⎤	
Triptafen	amitriptyline and perphenazine	Depression
Fluanxol	flupenthixol ⎦	
Depixol	flupenthixol ⎤	
Largactil	chlorpromazine	
Moditen	fluphenazine	Hallucinations
Haldol	haloperidol	Mild confusion or
Serenace	haloperidol	disorientation
Fentazin	perphenazine	Disturbed thinking
Orap	pimozide	
Melleril	thioridazine	
Stelazine	trifluoperazine ⎦	

Figure 7: Table of drugs to be avoided or questioned if they are prescribed

My brother has glaucoma. Does that mean that some Parkinson's drugs will not be available to him?

There is no major problem for people with glaucoma, especially if the glaucoma itself is being adequately treated. Anticholinergic drugs such as Artane will probably have to be avoided, but these Parkinson's drugs are not used very much now anyway. There is no problem with L-dopa replacement therapy (Madopar and Sinemet) or with dopamine agonists (all discussed earlier in this chapter). The drugs your brother needs for his glaucoma will not upset his Parkinson's.

Does having a pacemaker create any problems in Parkinson's medication?

There should be no problem with a pacemaker. In the days before L-dopa preparations included a dopa-decarboxylase inhibitor (ie before we had Sinemet and Madopar) there were some potential problems but not now. There is no problem with dopamine agonists either. When treatment for depression is also required, the cardiologist may, depending on the particular cardiac condition, be wary of some anti-depressant drugs.

Actually fitting and managing the pacemaker should cause no problems and cardiologists are well used to looking after people with other illnesses in addition to their heart complaints.

I have heard of people with Parkinson's having too much saliva but I have a dry mouth which I find very uncomfortable. Why should this be?

Yes, people with Parkinson's sometimes have too much saliva, not because more than normal is being produced, but because the continual swallowing which we all do is slowed down so the saliva accumulates in the mouth and can overflow. The dry mouth which you have is, however, likely to be related to your medication. This could either be an anticholinergic such as Artane or one of the anti-depressants. Changing the dosage may be helpful but you have, of course, been given these drugs for a good reason so you need to discuss the various options with your doctor. Once again it is a question of trying to find a fairly happy medium.

Sucking glycerine and honey sweets may help to make your mouth feel less dry, and ice cold water or citrus-flavoured drinks with or between meals can also be helpful.

Long-term problems

Why do some people with Parkinson's suffer from excessive movements of the head and body?

These are involuntary movements (as we mentioned in Chapter

2, they are also known as dyskinesias or choreiform movements). They vary greatly in their severity but are quite common, particularly in people who have had Parkinson's and been treated for it over a number of years. They are not well understood but seem to be part and parcel of artificially increasing the dopamine in the brain. We know that they are not just a side effect of the drugs because if people who do not have Parkinson's take these same drugs, they do not get these movements. They are partly caused by the Parkinson's and partly by the level of Madopar or Sinemet (there is a section about these drugs at the beginning of this chapter).

When involuntary movements appear, they are usually a sign that the dose of Madopar or Sinemet is on the high side, so a reduction in the dose is usually tried. However, this sometimes leads to a return of the Parkinson's symptoms of slowness and stiffness, and a new compromise between mobility and involuntary movements has to be sought.

The frequency and timing of the involuntary movements differs between individuals. In some, the movements are there most of the time, while in others they tend to appear just after taking a tablet or shortly before the next one is due. Some people find them very troublesome but, when they are fairly mild, they are often more upsetting to an observer than to the person with Parkinson's - as we discuss in the answer to the next question.

My son's involuntary movements distress me greatly and I think he should take fewer tablets but he disagrees. What do you think?

Other people often notice involuntary movements more - and are more disturbed by them - than the person with Parkinson's. Your son's argument will be that if he reduces the dose he will feel underdosed and his Parkinson's symptoms will return. In such a situation, particularly if his movements were severe, we would encourage him to try a reduction in the dose. If he tries and he does feel and look worse, you may have to accept that he is better off with the involuntary movements than without them.

Your son does need to understand that his involuntary movements are a sign that he is on the top dose of treatment that he can take (or even that he is already just over the top), so he should not just take more and more tablets thinking that they will help. The misconception that more is better can lead, in some people, to an obsession with their medication and when the next dose is due. Although this is understandable when people are experiencing severe fluctuations, it can sometimes lead to them taking more drugs that is sensible. Anyone who feels that their total daily dose of treatment is inadequate should discuss this with their doctor, and not simply increase the dose themselves.

My tablets do not seem to last as long as they used to so I have times, just before a dose, when I feel very slow and rigid. Why has this started to happen and what can be done to help?

What you are experiencing is fairly common after several years on L-dopa replacement therapy (which is discussed in the first section of this chapter). It is known as the 'wearing off' phenomenon for the obvious reason that the effectiveness of the medication 'wears off' before the next dose is due. There are various theories about why it happens but no satisfactory explanation at the moment. With drugs taken by mouth, the amount of the drug in the blood stream goes up and down fairly quickly but, in the earlier years of Parkinson's, the brain is able to handle these fluctuations and give a fairly smooth response. However, as the years go by the brain seems less able to do this and the benefit you get from your tablets starts to vary roughly in time with the level in the blood stream.

There are several possible ways of trying to improve the situation and you should talk to your doctor or specialist to see which one he or she recommends. There are three main options.

- Keep your total daily dose of Sinemet or Madopar about the same but take smaller doses more frequently.
- Take your tablets before, rather than with, meals so that the L-dopa has less competition from the protein in your food, and/or try redistributing your daily protein (eg meat, cheese,

eggs) so that most of it is taken at your evening meal rather than at midday, so minimising any disruption of your daytime activities. (Chapter 9 on *Eating and diet* includes more information about protein in your diet.)

- Consider changing to one of the controlled release forms of Madopar or Sinemet. They keep the levels in the blood stream more constant and can reduce the fluctuations, but most people find that they need a mixture of the controlled release and ordinary forms of the drug.

If none of these work for you, your specialist might consider trying dopamine agonist tablets or capsules (there are questions about these drugs earlier in this chapter). If this is the chosen option, it may be necessary to reduce your dose of the L-dopa preparation as otherwise you may start getting too many involuntary movements.

My wife has had Parkinson's for many years and now she can change from reasonable mobility to absolute immobility in minutes. What causes this sudden change?

Your question contains a very good description of something we call the 'on/off' phenomenon. Some people call it 'yo-yoing'. It usually happens with people (like your wife) who have had Parkinson's for five to 10 years or so. It is just as you describe, in that people can go from being quite well, with or without some involuntary movements, to becoming immobile, perhaps with recurrence of tremor, all in the space of a few minutes. This phase can last for quite some time and differs from the freezing (described in Chapter 2) which happens whilst walking and which lasts for seconds rather than minutes or hours.

The explanation of these fluctuations is, like the 'wearing off' phenomenon, not understood and is a major target for research. The current explanation is similar to that for the 'wearing off' phenomenon. In other words, as the years go by people become very sensitive to the amount of the drug in their blood stream and this triggers (sometimes very quickly) changes in symptoms from being 'on' (well and able to move around, with or without involuntary movements) to being 'off' (immobile with or without tremor).

Improving the situation is even more difficult than for the 'wearing off' phenomenon, although the same changes to treatment are usually tried (we have listed these in the answer to the previous question). Your wife's specialist may suggest that she tries an injected form of dopamine agonist called apomorphine (Britaject) rather than a tablet form. There is more about apomorphine in the section on **Dopamine agonists** earlier in this chapter.

My mother has great difficulty in swallowing and getting her tablets down is becoming a major problem. Can anything be done to help?

Swallowing can be a problem with Parkinson's although it is not very common and usually not severe. Because it is uncommon, especially in the early years, the doctor should check for other possible causes. You should certainly mention it to her doctor to see whether a further opinion from a throat specialist would be sensible. If your mother's problems turn out to be due to her Parkinson's, her medication could be reviewed. Anticholinergic drugs tend to cause a dry mouth which can exacerbate swallowing difficulties so, if she is taking any of these, her doctor might suggest gradually trying without them.

There are two other things that can be done. First of all, if she finds liquids easier to swallow than solids, there is a soluble form of Madopar called Madopar dispersible which can be dissolved in water. Some changes of dosage and timing may be necessary, and this will be explained by her doctor. There may be a short period of trial and error until she gets the same effect as with her previous tablets. The second line of attack is for her specialist or GP to consider involving a speech and language therapist. They have a special interest in swallowing and can often suggest ways of easing the problem.

There is some more information about swallowing problems in Chapter 9 on **Eating and diet**.

My elderly mother is constantly drooling. What can be done to help?

Having saliva overflowing from the mouth (some people call this drooling, others dribbling) is a problem which is quite common in advanced Parkinson's. It is not so much that more saliva is produced but that, without realising it, the natural tendency to swallow every now and again (even when not eating) is slowed down, so allowing an accumulation of saliva in the mouth. The saliva can then overflow, especially as good lip closure is more difficult for people with Parkinson's and there is also a tendency for the head to be bent forwards.

This can be a difficult problem to solve. The anticholinergic drugs (discussed earlier in this chapter) and some of the drugs used for depression can help but anticholinergic drugs tend to have quite a lot of undesirable side effects, especially in the elderly. The same drugs can be given by skin patches but tend to have the same side effects as the tablets and, in addition, may cause sore skin.

Very occasionally surgery or radiation therapy on the salivary glands has been attempted. Although this treatment has been known for many years, it is rarely used as the results are unpredictable and can cause side effects, including an over-dry mouth.

My husband who is in his seventies has been taking anti-Parkinson's drugs for many years. Lately, he has developed terrible nightmares and has hallucinations during the day – sometimes he maintains he can see soldiers marching through the room and so forth. Both of us find this very distressing. Can you explain what could be causing this and whether anything can be done to help?

Thank you for bringing up this problem which is not too uncommon, especially in people over the age of 70 who have had Parkinson's for a long time (as in your husband's case). As with many things that happen with Parkinson's, there is no simple explanation. We know that they are not just a side effect of the drugs because if people who do not have Parkinson's take these same drugs, they do not get hallucinations. The likely explanation is that they are partly caused by the Parkinson's and partly by the drugs.

Virtually any of the drugs used to treat Parkinson's can be

partly to blame. If your husband is on anticholinergics, most doctors would start by trying to reduce them, and then slowly stop them altogether. However, usually it is L-dopa replacement therapy or a dopamine agonist which is to blame. In some people reducing these drugs can get rid of the problem but this may be at the expense of increasing immobility. In this case a not very happy intermediate course has to be tried, aiming for reasonable mobility and some reduction in the hallucinations, but perhaps not eliminating them altogether. Although it sounds unlikely in your case, some people do not find their hallucinations or dreams particularly upsetting so, for them, these difficult compromises are not necessary. If, on the other hand, distressing hallucinations and confusion continue even after significant reductions in the drugs, it could, sadly, mean the onset of dementia.

Drugs that are given to treat hallucinations in other diseases unfortunately have a tendency to make the symptoms of Parkinson's worse, so your husband would not find them helpful. Research is taking place into new drugs that would avoid this problem, but they are still at the experimental stage and not yet available as a form of treatment.

Whatever the outcome of adjustments to your husband's drug regime, if you are not already receiving support and advice from your local health professionals, Social Services or from the Parkinson's Disease Society, we would strongly recommend that you seek out such help. You may also find some of the suggestions in the *Caring for the carers* section of Chapter 5 helpful.

Physical therapies

I recently had a course of physiotherapy after a fall due to my Parkinson's and found it a great help. No one ever suggested it before. Why is it not more widely available?

Physiotherapy is of use with Parkinson's although clearly it cannot correct the whole problem. Many people have had a similar experience to yours – they have found physiotherapy extremely helpful after a fall or when they have been made immobile, perhaps because of an operation. In these situations, physiotherapy helps people to get going again and restores any confidence which they may have lost. It is also quite helpful in people who are having difficulty with their walking.

Physiotherapy is not often recommended in the very early stages of Parkinson's, although there are some people (including one of the authors and several physiotherapists!) who think that an early referral for assessment and advice on exercises and self-help can have important, long-term advantages. Usually people are just advised by their doctors to keep as active as possible. In general we agree that referrals for physiotherapy are not made as often as they should be, partly because there is a shortage of physiotherapists but also because there is lack of awareness about how helpful their intervention can be. Sometimes it is necessary to be very persistent and nag your GP or specialist even to get a trial course to see whether it helps or not. Access to physiotherapy is discussed in Chapter 4 and there are more examples of the use of physiotherapy in Chapter 8.

One of the most frustrating aspects of my Parkinson's is the way it interferes with so many everyday tasks from doing up buttons to getting out of chairs and turning over in bed. What help can I get with these problems?

Certainly the problems which you describe are amongst the most frustrating and difficult aspects of Parkinson's. Although the medication usually helps considerably, it does not always provide the complete solution, and then help from both physiotherapists and occupational therapists can be very useful. Sometimes it is a case of finding a new way of tackling problems and sometimes a question of identifying the right type of equipment. You will find many examples of the ways these therapists can help in Chapter 8, and information about getting access to them in Chapter 4.

Can speech therapy help people with Parkinson's?

Speech therapy (now called speech and language therapy) can

be of benefit to some people with Parkinson's who are having problems with either their speech or their swallowing.

There can be a range of speech problems, from low volume and hoarseness to difficulty in getting started or speaking too quickly, and it is important to get the help of a speech and language therapist with an interest in Parkinson's. As with other therapists, speech and language therapists sometimes feel that they are brought in too late to have maximum effect. Even in the early stages they can suggest exercises which improve facial mobility and expressive speech and so help people retain good communication skills for longer than would otherwise be the case. There is more information on the ways in which they can help in Chapter 6 on *Communication*.

As we mentioned earlier in this chapter, speech and language therapists also have a special interest in swallowing and should be involved when this is causing problems. There is some more information about swallowing problems in Chapter 9 on *Eating and diet*.

How might a dietitian be involved in the treatment of Parkinson's?

There are several possibilities here. When people are having the severe involuntary movements or 'on/off' symptoms we discussed earlier in this chapter, one approach that can be taken is to reduce or rearrange the protein in their food. Such dietary changes are best undertaken with the advice of a dietitian. Secondly, people with Parkinson's can be overweight or underweight, and in both cases the advice of a dietitian may be sought. Finally, when there are swallowing problems, the dietitian can suggest ways of preparing and presenting food and drink so that it is both nutritious and easier to swallow (there are some suggestions about this in Chapter 9).

Surgical treatments

I have read that there used to be a surgical operation to

reduce severe tremor. Is this ever carried out now, and if not, why not?

The operation which you read about is known as stereotactic thalamotomy. It involves putting a very fine needle into the brain and causing careful and selective damage to certain cells in the thalamus. The thalamus is a part of the brain (located near the substantia nigra) which is responsible for relaying information from the sense organs about what is going on in the body to the various parts of the brain. The objective of the operation is to improve the tremor by 'circuit breaking' some overactive circuits within this part of the brain.

These operations were done quite often before drug treatment with L-dopa replacement therapy (Madopar and Sinemet) came along. They are rarely done now, especially as brain surgery always carries some risk. In any event, the drugs are thought to work better than the operations, although they are perhaps less effective against tremor than against slowness and rigidity. The operation was better, as you say, at reducing tremor which (although less disabling than slowness and rigidity) can be extremely embarrassing. It can only safely be done on one side as speech often deteriorates when it is done on both sides.

The operation is still considered when tremor on one side of the body is the chief problem and the tremor has not responded to medication. As few people fall into this category, the operation has become a rarity.

There seems to be renewed interest in another operation called pallidotomy. Can you explain what this involves? Is it likely to be helpful to some people with Parkinson's?

Palliditomy is another form of stereotactic surgery (see the *Glossary* for a definition of this term) which uses similar techniques to those described in the answer to the previous question to damage and so 'circuit break' some overactive circuits in a small area in another part of the brain called the pallidum. First carried out in the 1950s, it was rediscovered in the 1980s and results suggest that it may help all the main symptoms of Parkinson's (slowness, rigidity and tremor). To date most of the operations have been carried out in Sweden and the United States. Further research will help to establish which people and which symptoms are most responsive to this treatment and what the balance of advantages and disadvantages is likely to be. Although the procedure is still at the experimental stage, it is a promising development. We will have to be patient for a little longer before we can be more definite about its prospects.

I would like to know more about foetal cell transplantation surgery – can you give me some information?

Yes – we have discussed it in Chapter 13 on *Research and clinical trials*.

Complementary therapies

Do doctors disapprove of complementary or alternative medicines?

Before trying to answer this question, we need to make a distinction between medicines or therapies which claim to be 'alternatives' to the treatment offered by the medical profession, and those which are 'complementary' and are meant to be used alongside conventional treatments. The use of a complementary therapy should be in addition to, and not instead of, your usual treatment – no one should stop taking their normal drugs without a doctor's approval.

Doctors in general are happier with the idea of complementary therapies. The medical profession seems to be becoming more sympathetic to these therapies, some of which are very ancient, and is perhaps also more aware of the shortcomings in what it has to offer in some situations. At the same time, the reputable members of these various therapies are trying harder to improve their own practices and to give the public more information about their qualifications and training. The British Complementary Medicine Association and the Institute for

Complementary Medicine (see Appendix 1 for addresses) are useful sources of further information, or you can enquire at your own GP surgery or health centre for the names of reputable local practitioners. Some practices now offer certain complementary therapies themselves.

The reservations held by many members of the medical and health professions largely revolve around the fact that very few of these treatments have been subjected to properly controlled trials. This means that there is little hard evidence that the treatments really work. Efforts are being made to address this problem and there is now a Research Council for Complementary Medicine (address in Appendix 1), and the University of Exeter has the first Professor of Complementary Medicine in Europe.

Doctors get upset about alternative or complementary medicines when people are tempted to stop their normal treatment, when the therapies have serious side effects, and when they feel that their patients are being misinformed and persuaded to spend large sums of money which they can ill afford. If these features are not present, most practising doctors will take a benign view of these forms of therapy and appreciate that, even if the scientific evidence or rationale for them is elusive, they may well do some good. This is especially likely if the people concerned feel enthusiastic about them. They may give people a sense of doing something for themselves which can be very valuable and may also help them to relax.

I like the idea of music therapy. What does it have to offer people with Parkinson's?

Music therapy sounds delightful and certainly has no harmful side effects. Many people with Parkinson's discover for themselves that listening to strong rhythmic music can improve their walking, prevent hesitations, and overcome freezing episodes. Some find that they are still able to dance even though walking is difficult and that they tire less easily when moving to music. Music with a regular beat and perhaps a tune which is familiar or has some emotional significance seems to be the most helpful. The skilled music therapist can use music in a structured way to build on these observations. In this way, music therapy can help with physical activities like walking and upper limb movements, with involuntary movements and tremor, and with speech disturbances. It can also reduce fatigue. Music therapists often work on these problems with other therapists such as physiotherapists and speech and language therapists.

It is not necessary to have any musical experience to enjoy the benefits of music therapy. The benefits are most obvious during the therapy sessions, but preliminary studies suggest that there is a significant 'carry-over' effect.

Unfortunately music therapists are rather thinly spread across the United Kingdom and gaining access to them may be difficult. If you are interested, contact the Association of Professional Music Therapists (see Appendix 1 for the address) to see if there is one working in your part of the country.

Is hypnosis useful in overcoming Parkinson's symptoms such as tremor, 'off' periods and freezing?

We have probably all heard about the use of hypnosis in helping people break bad habits, such as smoking, and it is also sometimes used in illnesses which are thought to have a large psychological component (hypnosis is said to put you more in touch with your subconscious self). It may also help in conditions like Parkinson's which are aggravated by stress.

When you are hypnotised, you enter a state of very deep relaxation. People can be taught self-hypnosis, and some therapists may provide audiocassettes that you can listen to at home to help with this. In Parkinson's, it is most likely to help with stress management and in doing so help to reduce tremor, excessive sweating and, perhaps, involuntary movements. If it helps you to relax and cope with stress more effectively, it may also reduce the discomfort of 'off' periods and episodes of freezing.

If you feel that hypnosis might help you, discuss it with your GP who may be able to suggest a reputable practitioner. If this is not possible, follow the suggestions given in the first question in this section and consult one of the main complementary medicine organisations for advice.

Is there any evidence that homeopathy can help in Parkinson's?

To our knowledge, there is no good evidence that homeopathy can help in any very specific way. However, as with the other complementary therapies, it tries to look at the person as a whole and, in so doing, may lead to overall improvements in well-being.

Some people say that osteopathy can help with Parkinson's symptoms. Is this true?

We can't give a definite answer to this question, partly because there are no carefully controlled studies of its use in Parkinson's but also because many people with Parkinson's have other conditions which may respond to osteopathy. Certainly there are osteopaths who feel they have a contribution to make and people with Parkinson's who feel they have been helped. Many doctors accept that osteopathy can be helpful for the aches and pains to which people with Parkinson's are prone. It is important to find a registered osteopath (see Appendix 1 for address of the General Council and Register of Osteopaths, the largest of the regulating bodies). Osteopathy is to be the first complementary therapy to become a regulated profession (in the same way that doctors, nurses and dentists are regulated): eventually the General Council and the other regulating bodies will transfer their functions to a new governing body, to be called the General Osteopathic Council.

Would aromatherapy help my husband as he is in great discomfort in bed?

It is impossible to predict whether or not aromatherapy will help your husband. If his discomfort is due to inability to relax or to painful muscles and joints, it could be worth a try. It certainly seems to relax many people although whether this is the result of the massage or the oils themselves is difficult to establish. The oils can also be used in the bath, although this is thought to be somewhat less effective.

There is no doubt that the essential oils used in aromatherapy can be absorbed through the skin and that some of them have been in use for many, many years. Shirley Price (see Appendix 1 for the address of her company – Shirley Price Aromatherapy Ltd) is an aromatherapist with a special interest in Parkinson's who has recently carried out some small scale research using clary sage, sweet marjoram and lavender oils, and hopes to do more. She feels that it is most likely to help in improving movement ability and in reducing insomnia and constipation. She also emphasises that some commercially obtainable oils can be toxic for some people (it is important not to assume that because something is natural it is therefore safe) so you should consult a reputable therapist.

More conventional approaches which might also help your husband's problems are controlled release versions of Sinemet or Madopar, light sedatives and painkillers, or adjustments to his bedding or nightwear. Do discuss these possibilities – and that of aromatherapy – with his GP if you have not already done so.

My friend says that she has been helped a lot by yoga classes. How might this work?

We also know of people who have been helped by yoga. In its overall philosophy and its emphasis on mind over matter, it can give people a sense of purpose and of being in control of their lives. As it can improve people's ability to relax and to keep their joints and muscles mobile and supple, it is easy to see why it might help. It may also improve coordination and relieve some of the muscular aches and pains that are common with Parkinson's. Additionally, the wellbeing that many people feel after physical activity may help relieve anxiety or any tendency towards depression.

Yoga is, however, more a way of life than an occasional activity and requires quite a lot of commitment and self-discipline. Further information can be obtained from the Yoga for Health Foundation (see Appendix 1 for the address).

Are there any other complementary therapies that can help in Parkinson's?

There are many other complementary therapies from which

people with Parkinson's feel they have benefitted. In many cases people benefit because the therapy helps them to relax, or encourages them to exercise or to think positively. Whichever complementary therapy you choose, discuss your ideas with your doctor, check on the therapist's qualifications, and try to talk to other people with Parkinson's who have also tried that particular therapy. It is also a good idea to check what costs will be involved – complementary therapies are not usually available on the NHS and can be quite expensive.

4
Access to treatment and services

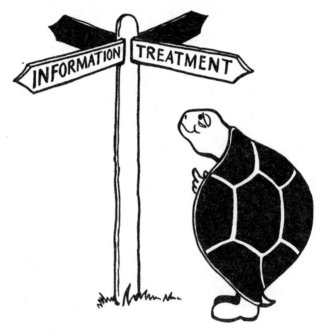

Introduction

When you need treatment or a particular service, it can be especially frustrating to be passed from pillar to post before discovering the appropriate person or organisation. This chapter addresses questions about access to professional services: we hope to make your search for help shorter and more effective. However, we need to add a word of caution. There has been a major reorganisation of health and social services since

1992, a reorganisation which is still progressing and which makes it particularly difficult for us to give definite answers to some questions. We will therefore try to outline what we believe to be the general or usual situation, but ask you to refer to organisations in your own local area for details of provision, entitlement and charging.

Medical treatment and related services

How can I find a consultant specialising in Parkinson's?

As Parkinson's is a neurological condition (a condition affecting the body's nervous system) the most appropriate specialist is a neurologist. You have to go through your GP who will know if there is a neurologist at your nearest hospital and, if not, where one is located. However as Parkinson's is mainly a disease which affects older people, some geriatricians (doctors specialising in the medical care of older people) are also very knowledgeable about it. The Parkinson's Disease Society (see Appendix 1 for their address) is able to provide the names of neurologists in your area but cannot recommend any particular ones.

Are there advantages in making a private appointment?

There may be – if you have private health insurance or if you can otherwise afford it – although the quality of care will not necessarily be better. Because there is a shortage of neurologists in this country, some of them have long waiting lists for first appointments and long gaps between follow-up appointments. You still need a referral from your own doctor but, by paying for a private appointment, you may be able to see the specialist more quickly. You can also be sure of seeing that particular person rather than another member of the medical team and you also tend to get rather more time with the specialist.

If money is not a problem, you can remain as a private patient and retain these advantages. However, it is important to remember that treatment is likely to continue for the rest of your life and that the cost may become a very heavy burden.

Many specialists will arrange a transfer to their NHS list for people who choose a private first appointment just to obtain a diagnosis and begin treatment.

In some places there are now NHS Parkinson's or neuro-care clinics which offer, in addition to medical consultation, access to other members of the health team such as Nurse Specialists, counsellors and therapists. Geriatricians also tend to have access to these other health workers so, in some circumstances, there could be advantages in **not** being a private patient.

I would like to see a specialist but my GP refuses to refer me. Can I insist?

There is a widely held belief that you have an absolute right to see a specialist but this is not so. What the *Patient's Charter* (see Appendix 2 for how to obtain a copy) promises is the right 'to be referred to a consultant acceptable to you **when your GP thinks it necessary** and to be referred for a second opinion if **you and your GP** agree this is desirable' (our emphasis).

In reality there are things you can do to increase your chances of being referred. It is helpful to explain fully to your GP why you feel a referral is necessary and to discover the reason for refusal. Usually a GP will think it is reasonable to have the diagnosis and management of Parkinson's confirmed by a specialist. Take a relative or friend with you if you feel that you need moral support or someone to speak for you.

If, having exchanged views, your doctor continues to say 'no' and you still want to pursue the matter, you could try changing your GP as a different one may be more sympathetic. However this cannot be guaranteed, and the pros and cons of such a move need to be carefully considered especially if, in general, you like your GP and the practice or it is conveniently situated. Although you have no right to be referred to a specialist, you do have a right to be registered with a GP and to change to another one without giving a reason. Your local Family Health Services Authority or your Community Health Council (their telephone numbers will be in your local phone book) can advise you about this.

I have seen a few news items about Parkinson's Nurse Specialists. What are they?

Nurse Specialists are a fairly new concept in nursing but they have emerged in several fields in recent years, most notably with the Macmillan Nurses who care for people with cancer. Other Nurse Specialists work with people who have diabetes, with people with asthma, with those who have bowel and bladder problems and – quite recently, as you note – with people with Parkinson's.

All Nurse Specialists have a general nursing training, plus training and experience in their chosen specialist field. Parkinson's Nurse Specialists have extensive knowledge about Parkinson's and the drugs used in its treatment, and they work closely with those who have Parkinson's, their carers and other health professionals.

If Parkinson's Nurse Specialists are such a new idea, does that mean that there are not very many of them around?

You are right: this is a very new idea. To give you some idea of numbers, there are currently five Nurse Specialists who are employed by the Parkinson's Disease Society in various parts of England and who work with hospital consultants (neurologists, geriatricians or physicians) in their areas. There are also 12 nurses who are employed by St Mary's Medical School in London, who will shortly be assigned to certain Health Authority areas to work with GPs. Both these groups of nurses are working in time-limited projects funded by money from the Parkinson's Disease Society, drug companies and individual donors. Their work will be studied carefully and the results published in medical and nursing journals. All Health Authorities will then have access to this evidence to help them to decide whether the Nurse Specialists should be funded by the Health Service and so become a more permanent part of health provision.

There are also some other individual Nurse Specialists working with people with Parkinson's in various centres around the United Kingdom. Most of these posts have been created through the enthusiasm and commitment of a local doctor, nurse or Parkinson's Disease Society branch. Sometimes these nurses work just with people with Parkinson's, sometimes with a wider group of people with neurological conditions.

So as you can see, as yet there are not many Parkinson's Nurse Specialists working in the National Health Service – but then a few years ago there were only a handful of diabetes or asthma specialist nurses, and now they are in posts all over the country. We very much hope that over the next few years we will see similar numbers of Parkinson's Nurse Specialists.

How can I get to see a Parkinson's Nurse Specialist?

For the nurses who are attached to one of the two time-limited projects, access is restricted to people whose doctors (consultants or GPs) are involved in the project. Some of the individual Nurse Specialists have more flexible referral arrangements. You can find out whether there is a Parkinson's Nurse Specialist in your area (and whether you need to be on a particular doctor's list) by contacting the Parkinson's Disease Society's National Office (address in Appendix 1).

Contacts with Parkinson's Nurse Specialists are usually at the clinic or GP's surgery, but can also include home visits when these are considered necessary. Depending on what other sources of help are available locally (for example, Parkinson's Disease Society welfare visitors), the Parkinson's Nurse Specialist may either concentrate on a particular problem such as drug management, or may be a more general source of advice, support and contact with other services.

I have read that exercise and physiotherapy are beneficial but my GP says physiotherapy won't help. What can I do?

The problem may lie in what is meant by 'help'. Your GP may mean that physiotherapy cannot cure Parkinson's and in that he or she is correct. However, you are also correct in thinking that, in most cases, exercise and physiotherapy can help by keeping your joints mobile and your muscles supple. Being more mobile and supple will mean that you feel more comfortable, and so more able to keep active and independent.

Of course the exercise needs to be appropriate for Parkinson's and for you personally. The simple exercises explained and illustrated in *Living with Parkinson's Disease* (see Appendix 2 for details of this booklet) were chosen by a physiotherapist and are well tried and tested.

Most NHS physiotherapy departments have waiting lists, and that may be one reason for your GP's reluctance to make a referral, but some departments do allow self-referrals so it would be worth contacting your local hospital or health centre to find out if this is possible. Some local branches of the Parkinson's Disease Society arrange group physiotherapy sessions (see Appendix 1 for the Society's address - they will tell you how to contact your nearest branch) and there are a growing number of private physiotherapists who run clinics and make home visits. If you choose private treatment, you will, of course, have to pay for this yourself and some physiotherapists may have little experience of treating Parkinson's. You also need to ensure that they are professionally qualified - look for the letters MCSP after their names. It could be worth having another discussion with your GP before deciding to start spending money!

I live in a remote country village and have had Parkinson's for 20 years. I urgently need dental treatment but have severe involuntary movements and can't find a dentist who will accept me. How can I obtain treatment?

Your first move should be to contact your Family Health Services Authority (it should be listed in your local phone book) and explain the difficulties you are having. They may know of a dentist who can treat you either in the surgery or at home. A dentist who can offer treatment under sedation (an injection given under the supervision of a doctor after which you remain conscious but relaxed) might be appropriate. If the Family Health Services Authority cannot help, you can contact the British Society of Dentistry for the Handicapped (see Appendix 1 for the address and telephone number). They keep a list of dentists interested in treating people with Parkinson's and would try to identify someone for you. Another option might be referral by your dentist or doctor to a dental hospital where in-patient treatment, perhaps under anaesthetic, could be provided.

Living in a remote village is an extra complication but all people with Parkinson's need to take care of their teeth or dentures and to keep their mouths in a healthy condition. This is especially true if they suffer from dryness in the mouth.

My elderly mother needs her eyes retesting but I don't drive and she is very difficult to move. Could I get someone to come and see her at home?

Yes. Many opticians will now do home visits to people who are housebound. If you have any difficulty finding one who will visit your mother at home, contact your Family Health Services Authority (the telephone number should be in your local phone book) and ask them to help you identify a suitable optician. If your mother is entitled to a free NHS sight test this service will be free but otherwise a charge will be made.

My speech is becoming less distinct and very hoarse and quiet. I think a speech therapist may be able to help. Can I refer myself or do I need to go through my doctor?

You are wise to consider getting a proper assessment of your speech difficulties and a speech therapist (or speech and language therapist as they are now called) is the best person to do this. Although most health districts suffer from a shortage of speech and language therapists, there are a growing number who have an interest in Parkinson's, so you should certainly ask (and if necessary persist in asking) to see one. You can refer yourself by contacting the Speech and Language Therapy Department at your local hospital or health centre, but because of the changing funding arrangements in the NHS, you will have a better chance of getting this service if you get a referral from your GP.

Speech and language therapists can also help with swallowing problems if these occur.

Doing various tasks around the house is becoming more difficult and, as my husband is also disabled, I feel we need some good advice about what to buy, etc. Who could do this?

There are many aids and appliances which can make household tasks more manageable but you are very wise to seek advice first, as it is easy to spend money on things which are not suitable or which are unduly expensive. The person who can help is the occupational therapist and you should ask your GP to refer you. Some occupational therapists work from a hospital or from Community Health Services and others from Social Services departments (there is a section on *Social Services and Community Health Services* later in this chapter).

Sometimes the solution is not a piece of equipment but rather a new way of organising your work space or of approaching a task, and occupational therapists are very skilled in these matters. The therapist may be able to lend you equipment to try out at home or, alternatively, may arrange a visit to one of the Disabled Living Centres (see Appendix 1 for the Disabled Living Centres Council's address – they will give you details of your nearest centre) where you can see and try some of the bigger and more expensive items.

If the occupational therapist decides that adaptations like rails or ramps are required, then he or she can make a recommendation to the appropriate Social Services department. There are many variations between areas in the charges made for these aids to daily living and, if you are worried about the possible costs, be sure to mention this to the therapist.

My walking, even around the house, is not good but part of the problem is my feet which I am now unable to care for properly. How can I obtain chiropody services?

Comfortable feet are very important for mobility and independence and many people, especially those who are elderly, need access to chiropody services. You should enquire at your GP's surgery or at the Community Health Services about the chiropody services available in your area. Most Community Health Services run clinics and have a domiciliary (home visiting) service for people with mobility problems so you should be able to arrange regular appointments. (You will find more information about Community Health Services later in this chapter.)

There are also private chiropodists if you are able to pay. If you do decide to see a chiropodist privately, make sure that he or she is State Registered (they will have the letters SRCh after their name).

I know that people with Parkinson's are advised to eat a balanced diet with plenty of fluids and high-fibre foods but this is difficult for me because of a chronic bowel condition. Could I get some additional advice from a dietitian?

You are quite right about the general dietary advice given to people with Parkinson's (see Chapter 9 for further questions on this topic) but also wise to realise that there can be exceptions to any general rule. First you should talk to your GP or specialist about the ways in which Parkinson's and your bowel condition could affect each other. You could also explain that you want to help yourself by eating sensibly and, if the doctor is not able to offer you enough guidance, you could ask for a referral to a dietitian. Most dietitians work in hospitals but an increasing number are working in the community, and in some places you can approach them directly without going through your GP.

My elderly father has prostate trouble as well as advanced Parkinson's and is now incontinent at night. Who can I ask for help with the psychological and practical problems this causes?

We assume that everything possible has been done to investigate and treat the incontinence problem. If not, you should contact your father's GP and ask for this to be done as soon as possible. You should also ask his GP to refer him to the local Continence Adviser or district nurse who will assess his needs and provide advice, support and practical guidance about obtaining pads, pants and laundry services. There is also a confidential advice line run by the Continence Foundation which you can use (see Appendix 1 for the address and telephone number).

Social Services and Community Health Services

My elderly mother is going to come and live with me as she can no longer cope alone. How can I find out what care services are available in my area?

You should contact the Social Services department and the Community Health Services for the area in which you live. They have a duty to provide information about their services and about which people are eligible for them. They should also provide information about any charges which you may incur.

We discuss what is offered by Social Services departments and Community Health Services in more detail in the answers to the next few questions.

What services do Social Services departments provide?

Social Services departments are part of local authorities and are responsible for providing services to people with various social and welfare needs. People who are elderly or who have a physical, mental or learning disability form the majority of their clients. Social Services departments provide (or increasingly nowadays arrange access to) places in luncheon clubs, day centres and residential homes; practical help in the home such as home helps, home care workers and Meals on Wheels; and adaptations and special equipment which enable people to stay in their own homes. Social Services departments also provide information, advice and counselling to people who are old or disabled and to their carers (see Chapter 5 for further discussion of services for carers).

What is the difference between home helps and home care workers?

It is difficult to be dogmatic about this and we suspect that there is still considerable overlap between the two roles, but basically home helps undertake cleaning in addition to other tasks whereas home care workers tend to concentrate on personal care (and may be forbidden to clean). Personal care can involve help with getting washed and dressed, getting to the toilet and preparing meals (see Chapter 8 for more questions on these topics).

I have heard people talking about Community Health Services. What exactly do they provide?

Community Health Services (often now organised into Community Health Trusts) are part of the National Health Service and they provide health services in people's own homes or in health centres. These services include district nurses, health visitors, community psychiatric and mental handicap nurses, psychologists, physiotherapists, occupational therapists, speech and language therapists, dietitians and chiropodists. Some Community Health Services also provide advice and practical help on specific topics such as incontinence, cardiac care, mastectomy and colostomy. You should be able to obtain access to most of the services mentioned above through your GP or practice nurse even if, in some areas, certain services are organised through the hospital rather than through the Community Health Services.

My wife is becoming increasingly disabled with Parkinson's and I have a heart condition. I have been told that we could be eligible for a community care assessment – what does this entail?

Since April 1993 every Social Services department has been required by law to have a coordinated system for assessing the needs of vulnerable people in the community. In order to request an assessment, all you have to do is to contact your local Social Services department either directly or through your doctor or other professional worker. (In some areas there is a .backlog of assessments, so you may meet delays and some persistence may be required!)

You will then be asked about your needs and if they cannot be met by the provision of a particular service like home care, but seem rather complex (as they could well be when there are two people with health problems) then an assessor will be assigned to you. He or she will make more detailed enquiries and will coordinate reports from any professionals with relevant knowledge or experience. The aim is to try to fit the services to the client rather than (as often happened in the past) vice versa and to ensure that you do not have to apply separately to lots of different departments to have your needs assessed.

Two other important characteristics of community care assessments are that the professionals involved are obliged to take account of your views and also to consider the needs of the carer. In your case – and in several others we have encountered – it is not always clear who is caring for whom! If your needs are agreed to be complex and they fall within the criteria established by your Social Services department, a care manager will be assigned to you (see the answer to the next question for more about care managers).

Every Social Services department has to publish information about its Community Care arrangements so you could telephone your local department and ask for a leaflet. These leaflets should also be available in your library, community centre or GP's surgery.

What is a care manager?

A care manager is the person from Social Services (or sometimes from Community Health Services) who is given the task of putting together, monitoring and reviewing the plan of care agreed after a community care assessment (discussed in the answer to the previous question). You should be given a copy of this plan and if you disagree with what is suggested, your disagreement should be recorded in writing.

If you feel that the plan fails to meet some of your needs, it is important to make this clear and to ask that the plan be reconsidered. Do feel free to involve a relative, friend or voluntary worker if you are in need of moral or practical support. If none of these people are available to you, ask the social worker or the local Citizens' Advice Bureau, Council for Voluntary Service or Community Health Council (all the addresses and telephone numbers should be in your local phone book) to help you to find an advocate, that is someone to help you put your point of view.

My mother is nearly blind and my father has Parkinson's. We have asked for a home care worker and someone to help them have a bath but Social Services say they cannot help. Surely they have to help us?

Without knowing more details, it is difficult for us to judge but it certainly sounds as though you have a case for a proper assessment of your parents' needs (and yours too in so far as you are a carer). Please read the earlier question and answer about community care assessments. If your mother is almost blind and is not registered as blind or partially sighted, arranging such registration through her local Social Services should improve her access to several services and benefits. Your parents' overall needs will depend on how disabled your father is (people with Parkinson's can be quite capable if their medication is well-balanced and they look after themselves in other ways). As explained in an answer earlier in this section, home care workers are sometimes forbidden to do housework and, if that is what your parents need, it may be better to try to find someone privately.

Help with bathing is another issue on which there is considerable controversy, and much variation in provision from place to place. In some areas Community Health Services provide a bathing service through nurses or bathing assistants, whereas in others this is not available. Another problem arises because of different definitions of 'need'. Your father may feel unable to bathe your mother even though he is physically capable of doing so or she may find his help unacceptable. This kind of psychologically or emotionally based need may not be acknowledged by Social Services as 'real', but if it is a factor in your parents' situation, you should press your case and see if you can get some support from relevant local voluntary organisations which may know of other similar cases.

My mother lives alone but is finding the stairs very difficult to manage. What options does she have to maintain her independence?

There are many different options depending on her wishes, her income, the house's potential for adaptation and the services available locally from the Social Services and Housing departments.

First you need to sit down with her and discuss what she really wants to do. If her current home is suitable in every aspect except the stairs, then she could decide to live downstairs (if there is space and ground floor toilet and washing facilities) or she could consider having a stairlift installed. She can apply to the Social Services department to see if she meets their eligibility criteria for this service and, if she does, the social worker will explain when the lift can be supplied (there is sometimes a waiting list) and how much it will cost. The cost will depend on your mother's income. Her chances of being judged eligible for the service will be greater if the provision of a stairlift will substantially improve her chances of retaining her independence. If she is not eligible through Social Services or if there is likely to be an unacceptably long delay, she could decide to purchase a stairlift herself if she has sufficient funds. Before considering this option, she should get some advice from Social Services about which makes and models are considered appropriate and whether there is a reputable source of second-hand lifts (which cost much less than new ones).

If there seem to be advantages in moving to another house, either to be nearer to sources of help or because her current house has other disadvantages apart from the stairs, she can consider applying for rehousing or selling up and buying a more suitable property. Most areas now have a variety of specialised accommodation for older people offering different levels of supervision and/or support. The local Housing department should be able to tell her what is available in the area and what her chances of being allocated certain kinds of accommodation would be. The following questions and answers have some more information about this.

I own a small terraced house but am finding it difficult to manage. Can I apply to the Council for rehousing?

Yes, you can certainly approach your local authority Housing department about any housing problem whether you own your present accomodation or not. The options which will be open to you will depend on the severity of the problems you are facing, local housing resources, the demand for the type of housing you need, and the financial and other conditions which are attached to any such rehousing.

We see quite a lot in the papers about sheltered housing. What exactly does it mean and who owns it?

Sheltered housing is accommodation which is purpose-built for people who need a certain amount of supervision because of old age or disability, but who wish to maintain a home of their own. The amount of supervision available can vary from a warden on site who can be contacted in an emergency to high-dependency units where there is still a degree of privacy and independence, but where higher staffing levels allow assistance with meals and personal care. Sheltered housing may be owned by the local authority, by housing associations or by private companies and may be managed by various combinations of these organisations. Your local Housing department will be able to provide further information.

Questions about residential and nursing homes are discussed in the section on *Long-term care* in Chapter 12.

5
Attitudes and relationships

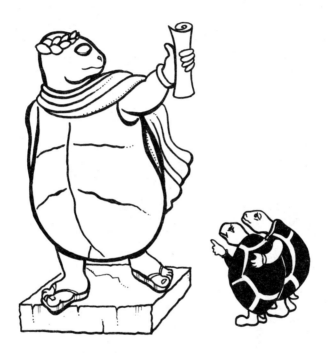

Introduction

Parkinson's is a real, physical illness but that does not mean that your attitude to it and the attitudes of other people that you encounter will make no difference. On the contrary, attitudes can make a big difference to how you feel about yourself and to how you try to make the best of your life with Parkinson's. Sidney Dorros, an American who did much to help other people with Parkinson's by writing about his own experiences, liked to talk of 'accommodation without surrender' and would remind people of an old saying – 'If you get a lemon, make lemonade'.

This chapter is also about the relationships – familial, professional and public – which impinge on people with Parkinson's and those who live with them or look after them. As will become clear, much can depend on the attitudes established in the early weeks and months after diagnosis and on people's willingness to talk through their difficulties and, if necessary, ask for help. There are also questions in this chapter about the needs of carers as these are closely linked with attitudes and with the relationships between the people with Parkinson's and their carers.

You and your partner

I have just been diagnosed with Parkinson's. It's a shock but I'd like to think there's something I can do to help myself. Is there?

Yes, there are lots of things you can do and you are already helping yourself by having such a positive attitude. If you think constructively about what you **can** do and how you can avoid and solve problems, you are already giving yourself a very good chance of coping well with Parkinson's. This does not mean that you will feel on top of things every day but that, in general, you will be looking for solutions rather than dwelling on problems.

Retaining your interests and activities (or replacing lost ones with something new), learning to maintain a good posture and doing suitable exercises (see Chapter 8) and eating sensibly (see Chapter 9) are all things that only you can do. Many people are also helped by gathering information about Parkinson's and its treatment (see Chapters 1 to 3) so that they understand better what is happening to them and how things work. Finally you can continue as you have started by being willing to ask questions and so being really involved in planning your own care.

I have just been diagnosed and don't want to tell my wife and family. What do you think I should do?

As we don't know you or the other members of your family, we can't give you specific advice but we can offer some ideas and questions for you to consider.

First you could try thinking through the consequences of telling or not telling your wife and family. If they know that you have been having some problems and that you have consulted the doctor, they will be expecting some information about the outcome. They will also have their own thoughts and fears and you will not know whether these are more or less distressing than a diagnosis of Parkinson's. Even quite small children can sense when something is wrong and pretending otherwise will not necessarily reassure them.

The other problem with not telling the truth is that the secret can come between you and your loved ones and create barriers where there were none before. You may also be depriving yourself of a very important source of help and comfort. However you may have some special reason for not 'telling' just yet, either because you are not feeling ready to talk about it or because one or more of your family are having some difficulties of their own just now.

It might be worth you talking the pros and cons over with a friend or counsellor. If you have no obvious source of help available locally, you could perhaps try the Parkinson's Disease Society's telephone Helpline (see Appendix 1 for the phone number). You will have to weigh the arguments for and against telling your wife and family but do remember that the task may seem to get bigger the longer you leave it.

I am 47, divorced but with a wonderful girlfriend. We had planned to marry but I have now been told I have Parkinson's. I don't know whether to go ahead with our plans or not.

If you have read Chapters 1 and 2 of this book you will know just how variable the impact of Parkinson's can be and how impossible it is to know what the future holds for any one individual. We do know that life expectancy is not very different from the normal and that many people cope well and have satisfying lives for many years.

Clearly you will have to talk to your girlfriend and you will both need to be honest about how you feel. You could perhaps go together to speak to your neurologist or GP, and friends or relatives could perhaps provide individual opportunities for you both to mull things over with a sympathetic listener. Alternatives might be your local branch of Relate (the former Marriage Guidance Council) who should be listed in your local phone book, or the Parkinson's Disease Society's Helpline or counsellor. (The Helpline phone number and the address of Relate's head office are given in Appendix 1.)

My husband, diagnosed earlier this year, gets tired easily. Should I encourage him to rest as much as possible?

No. Although it is true that fatigue is a common and often underestimated symptom of Parkinson's, it is also important that your husband keeps as active and involved in things as possible. If he becomes more dependent on you than is necessary, he will tend to feel helpless and bored, will have fewer topics to talk about and may become more liable to depression. In addition you will become more tied to the house and less able to keep up your own activities and interests, so both of you will suffer. One possible solution is to encourage your husband to do things for himself at times when he is at his best and to rest in between if necessary. If he rests too much during the day, his sleep at night may be affected, so creating another problem.

One of the big difficulties for relatives of people with Parkinson's is knowing when to encourage them to do things for themselves and how to recognise the times when this is not possible. As abilities can vary from day to day - and even from hour to hour - this task is not easy and requires great patience and sensitivity. Try to get other family members to understand how to keep this balance too. Don't be too discouraged if you don't always get it right. It **is** difficult and people don't become saints just because they or their spouses develop Parkinson's!

I'm a hyperactive, rather impatient person and I'm feeling

really bad about the way I snap at my wife who has Parkinson's and is therefore slower than she used to be. What can I do to make things easier for both of us?

Your question is a courageous and honest effort to face up to a difficult problem. As indicated in the answer to the previous question, people who develop Parkinson's, and their partners and families, do not stop being the people they were before. The challenge is to find a new way of living which takes account of all the elements in the new situation.

Perhaps the best way for you and your wife to start is to sit down together and acknowledge the problem and your sadness that you sometimes hurt each other. If you think her slowness has got worse recently, you could check with her GP or consultant whether any adjustment to her medication might help. Meanwhile you can try to identify the particular situations which you both find most frustrating and plan ways of avoiding or easing them. You may not realise, for example, that trying to hurry people with Parkinson's can make them slower, not faster. Both of you need to allow plenty of time for the tasks you intend to tackle so you have to accept the need for much more planning in your lives. One person with Parkinson's told us that this was, for him, the hardest thing to accept so we are not suggesting that it is easy! Having allowed enough time (and, where possible, having programmed activities for a part of the day when your wife is at her best), don't stand around and watch while your wife gets dressed, etc unless she needs your active assistance – go and do something else!

An extension to this last point is that you both need to retain or acquire some enjoyable activities which you can pursue independently of each other. Then, when you are together, you may find that you are able to be more relaxed and patient.

We have a very happy marriage, perhaps partly because we've always had some individual as well as shared interests. Now my husband has got Parkinson's and I'm afraid I will resent having to give up my own 'space'. Am I being selfish?

Your fears are very understandable and probably not selfish at all. Most doctors and other professionals involved with people who have been recently diagnosed stress the need for both parties to maintain their interests and independence and to live as normal a life as possible. Because Parkinson's can be difficult to diagnose, some people have been through many months of anxiety and uncertainty by the time that they get the diagnosis and treatment can begin. This can mean that they have already withdrawn a bit from their activities and their partner has had to do the same. However, once your husband has the correct treatment, you should both be able to pick up all or most of your earlier interests. As you suggest, such diversity can actually strengthen a marriage and it can certainly make any necessary adjustments which follow the onset of Parkinson's easier to handle.

I don't know how much longer I can cope. My husband was the dominant, decision-making partner in our marriage and we both liked it that way. Now he is quite disabled with Parkinson's but the real problem is that neither of us seem to be able to adjust to our new roles – I feel overwhelmed and indecisive and he feels frustrated and angry.

Every marriage or relationship is unique and there are many different ways of sharing the roles and being happy. The problems arise, as you have discovered, when circumstances change and your particular solution no longer works. We can't tell from your question whether you have felt able to sit down and talk these matters over with your husband. If you haven't, that would be the place to start. Outside help – from a trusted friend, from a counsellor (at the Parkinson's Disease Society or from a local source) or from an organisation like Relate may also enable you both to explore whether the situation can be improved and, if so, how. (If Relate is not listed in your local phone book, you can contact their head office at the address given in Appendix 1.)

I am 36, have recently been diagnosed as having Parkinson's and am beginning to understand some of the symptoms and

also what can be done to help. The thing that worries me most is how it might affect my relationship with my husband. This is a very understandable concern and it is a good sign that you can put your anxieties into words. Perhaps you will be able to take the next step and talk it over with your husband – you will probably find that he has some anxieties about this too.

'Relationships' within marriage have many aspects including the way in which roles are shared as well as specifically emotional and sexual aspects. Almost everything that happens to a couple can impinge on their emotional and sexual relationships and there is no doubt that Parkinson's can call for quite a lot of adjustments. There are very close links between how people feel about themselves and how satisfied they feel with their marital/sexual relationships. Because any illness or disability can affect our self-image, it can also affect our most intimate relationships, but we have reason to believe that many people with Parkinson's continue to have satisfactory marital and sexual relationships.

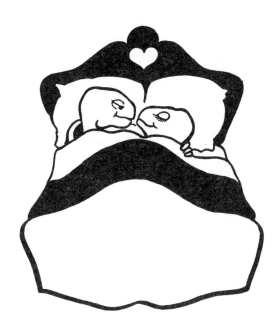

If it is the sexual aspects which cause you particular concern, there is a pamphlet called *Parkinson's Disease and Sex* (available from the Parkinson's Disease Society – details in Appendix 2) which has a clear and straightforward discussion of the nature of sexual function and sexual problems as well as information gathered from a group of people with Parkinson's. Those most likely to report problems were the couples in which the man had Parkinson's. Stress, anxiety and depression seemed to be more important causes of problems than anything directly related to the Parkinson's and something can usually be done to help in such circumstances.

One important piece of advice offered by several people with Parkinson's is to retain and treasure the small signs of affection and togetherness – touches, cuddles, kisses – which remind both the person with Parkinson's and the carer that they are lovable and loved.

Does Parkinson's cause impotence? My husband has become impotent at the age of 39, four years after being diagnosed.

Parkinson's can cause impotence as can the stress and anxiety which are sometimes associated with it. Some drugs used for other conditions may also have this side effect. If your husband has not already sought help, you should talk to him about the problem and encourage him to do so. His GP or neurologist may be able to help by referring him to someone with special expertise in this field.

Emotional support and counselling may be enough but, if not, there are other options which can be tried. For example, it has been shown that the injection of a drug called papaverine directly into the penis can sometimes be helpful. It leads to an erection and in people who have become impotent the result is often good enough to make this an acceptable and effective form of therapy. This is only one option, and there are others, so it is essential to get a correct diagnosis in order to ensure appropriate therapy.

You and your husband may also find that the pamphlet referred to in the previous question is helpful. There is an organisation called SPOD (Association to Aid the Sexual and

Personal Relationships of People with a Disability) which offers
help and advice (their address is in Appendix 1).

Does Parkinson's have any effect on fertility?

For obvious reasons, the number of people with Parkinson's who
are at the childbearing stage of life is very small, but we know of
both men and women with Parkinson's who have produced
children after they have been diagnosed.

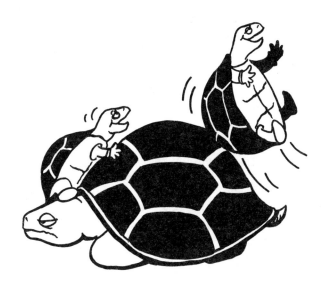

Children and grandchildren

**I am 38 and was recently diagnosed with Parkinson's. The
treatment is working well and only a few tell-tale symptoms
remain. We have two young children aged 4 and 2 and my wife
and I can't decide what to tell them. What do you think?**

Obviously your children are too small for complicated explana-
tions, but as in our answers in the previous section about the
pros and cons of telling family members, we think that honesty

is usually the best policy. With small children, who can be very sensitive to anxiety in their parents, you can just answer their questions as they arise or explain simply why you are tired or unsteady or whatever.

The Parkinson's Disease Society has commissioned some research into the needs of the children of people with Parkinson's and is planning to publish some books for children in different age groups.

My husband has had Parkinson's for nearly 20 years and is now quite disabled but he does love to have our grandchildren come to visit. However most of them live some distance away and can be quite daunted by his appearance and his mobility problems. What can we do to make their visits easier and more enjoyable for everyone?

You can encourage your children to visit at times when your husband is likely to be at his best and therefore more able to talk and listen and play. When his medication is working most effectively, his expression and mobility are likely to be less daunting to the grandchildren. A bit of explanation beforehand to the children about grandad's illness and the way that it hides 'the real grandad' may also help. Try to think of enjoyable and novel things to do while they are with you but do not allow the visits to be overlong. If your children or grandchildren want to help in some way, let them. Most of us feel more comfortable when we are being useful.

My wife is now very immobile and I often have to ask our teenage daughter to help me lift her or to stay in while I am working late. She is devoted to her mother but I don't want to take away her youth. How can I balance all our needs?

This is a difficult and sensitive problem. If you are convinced that everything possible has been done to maximise your wife's mobility, then you need to sit down together and discuss what options you have for rearranging your daily and weekly routines. Much will depend on what kind and quantity of help, from family and friends or from statutory and voluntary services, is available to you. It sounds as though a thorough, multi-disciplinary assessment (involving medical, nursing, therapy and Social Services personnel) would help and you can request this through your GP or Social Services department.

It is certainly wise to ensure that your daughter is able to spend time with her friends and to have leisure activities suited to her age, but she may also enjoy, and benefit from, the time she spends with her mother and feel good about being able to help. You don't say whether you also have a son. If you do, you should try to share the caring tasks between them rather than assume that these are girls' jobs. Most people find some caring tasks easier to cope with than others. It would be worth trying to discover if there are tasks such as toileting or bathing which your daughter or your wife find particularly distressing. You could then feed this information into the assessment process.

The Carers National Association (see Appendix 1 for their address) has a special worker with responsibility for young carers and they also produce an information pack (free to young carers) which you might find helpful.

My husband has had Parkinson's for many years but we have managed to keep up a normal family life and the children have taken the few necessary adjustments in their stride. Now one is 14 and discipline is becoming a problem. Some of the rows have been particularly hurtful to my husband. Is there anything we can do to improve matters?

Coping with adolescence creates problems for most families and there are no easy answers. You may find that talking things over with other couples, who are not also coping with a disabling illness, helps to put things in perspective. Talking among yourselves, acknowledging feelings on all sides and exploring how to avoid or cope better with the 'trigger' situations may also help. You may want to consider contacting YAPP&RS, the special section of the Parkinson's Disease Society for younger people. There are sure to be people there who have experienced similar problems.

If none of this seems sufficient, you could speak to the counsellor at the Parkinson's Disease Society (address and telephone number in Appendix 1). One small consolation is that adolescent problems tend to cure themselves in time.

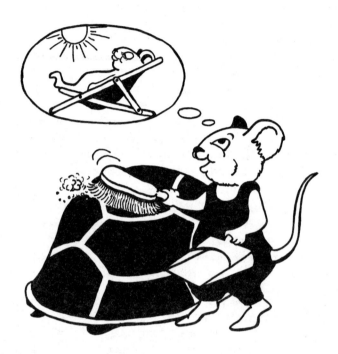

Caring for the carers

I have lived all my life with my mother who has Parkinson's and we are good friends as well as mother and daughter. I suppose that I am her 'carer' but I don't really like the word.

We understand your ambivalence about this word and your difficulty in applying it to yourself. In fact most of us resent being reduced to any one 'label' and fight to retain our many different facets. However the increased use of the word 'carer' has coincided with a growing awareness, among professionals and the general public, of the needs of people like yourself and, in general, that has been a very good thing. Parkinson's usually lasts for many years and, however good the relationship, it can bring limitations to the person who is caring as well as to the person with Parkinson's. It is helpful to both parties if carers have some time to themselves so that they can follow their own interests and recharge their batteries.

Our message would therefore be - yes, you are much more than a carer but don't let that fact stop you from taking advantage of any emotional, practical or financial help which is available.

I have been looking after my wife for 22 years. Mostly I don't mind the work or the responsibility but I do hate being taken for granted. Just occasionally I would like someone to ask about me.

We are sure that your words sum up the feelings of many people who look after their spouses or other relatives. In fact, when a group of people caring for their Parkinson's relatives got together to discuss their needs, recognition and acknowledgement were at the top of their list. To be told that you are doing a good job, to be asked for your opinion or to receive a caring enquiry about your own health and spirits can be a real boost.

Quite a lot of training for doctors, nurses, therapists and home carers is now including this sort of message and many trainers are discovering that the best people to deliver the message are people like yourself, who know what it is like to be a carer, 24 hours a day, seven days a week.

To return to the topic of your need to have someone, sometimes, ask about how you are feeling. We wonder if your own health is causing you some concern and, if so, would urge you to consult your doctor for a check-up. Carers often neglect themselves because they are so busy looking after their partner or relative, but in the long run, it is much better for both parties if the carer's health is properly supervised.

I am 55, fit and competent and very happy to care for my husband who is older than I am and who has had Parkinson's for many years. What riles me is the struggle to obtain proper information about the services and benefits which are

available – I can spend hours on the phone trying to locate the right office or person.

You are right to identify accurate and accessible information as a prime need of carers and to underline the stress and frustration which you experience when it is not available. It is unfortunately the case that in some instances what should be easily available in fact requires great persistence. The Carers National Association (see Appendix 1 for their address) has been in the forefront of campaigns to improve the situation and has, in addition to its national literature, helped to produce information guides called *Carers' A to Z* in many different parts of the country. Ask at your local Social Services, library or Health Centre to discover whether there is one for your area.

Access to information should also be improving in all areas as a result of the requirements of the Community Care Act. This requires Social Services departments to provide information about the services available in their locality and also to take account of the needs of carers when carrying out community care assessments (see Chapter 4 for information about obtaining access to a wide range of treatments and services). Some Social Services departments also have carers' support officers.

Another approach to ensuring that the carers of people with long-term illnesses have ready access to information is the allocation of a key worker to whom they can turn for information or advice. This system is being tried in some places and has much to recommend it.

The Parkinson's Disease Society has had several very successful Carers' Days in different parts of the country in recent years and is planning to publish a carers' handbook in the near future.

My wife is now very disabled and can't turn over or get in and out of bed without help. I am exhausted and feel in need of a rest. Could we get a night sitter?

'A good night's rest' was one of the needs of the group of Parkinson's carers that we mentioned in an earlier answer in this section and you certainly sound in need of just that. Some Community Health Services and Social Services departments have a night sitting service, although it is often pretty limited.

However, do ask at your GP's surgery or telephone Community Health Services (see your phone book for the number). Private sitters are also available but tend to be rather costly and you need to be sure that they are reputable. Again Community Health Services should have some information.

We wonder if you have also explored other ways of easing the situation. Night-time problems can sometimes be eased by changes in medication, so if you have not already discussed this with your wife's doctor we would urge you to do so. A physiotherapist can also help with advice for both the person with Parkinson's and their carer (see Chapter 8 for further discussion of this topic). Do ask your GP for a referral if you have not had access to such advice before.

There are other ways of arranging some respite for yourself and you will find examples of these in the answer to the next question and in Chapter 12 on *Care outside the home*.

My 80-year-old mother is now very frail and requires constant supervision. I am single and have no brothers or sisters so feel trapped in the house and more and more stressed. Can you suggest any solution?

All carers need some time for themselves if they are to continue being able to care, and you have obviously tried to manage without such help for too long. Approach your Social Services department and ask them to assess your needs as a carer (as well as your mother's) and say that you would like someone to come in and stay with your mother once or twice a week. Some Social Services departments now have contracts with a wonderful organisation called Crossroads Care whose objective is to give people like you a break. If you have a local Crossroads scheme you could also approach them direct (see your phone book for a local number, or Appendix 1 for the addresses and telephone numbers of the two national organisations, which are the Association of Crossroads Care Attendant Schemes and the Crossroads Scotland Care Attendant Schemes).

If these solutions are not available, try the nearest branch of the Parkinson's Disease Society (see Appendix 1 for the address of the national society who will be able to locate your nearest branch). They may be able to suggest other possible sources of sitters and also provide general support and advice to make your life a little easier.

My wife has had Parkinson's for over 20 years and I have no problems coping with the physical tasks of caring. However she has recently become quite confused and sometimes does not recognise me. I find this very distressing and would appreciate some practical and emotional support.

Support for the carers of people suffering from confusion and dementia (the general name for an illness in which the brain cells die faster than they do in normal ageing) is absolutely essential because, as you say, it is so distressing. However, first you must ensure that your wife's new symptoms are not due to some other temporary cause like infection, medicines or some other illness, so ask your doctor about this as soon as possible.

If the doctor decides that the cause of your wife's deteriorating mental abilities is dementia, you can obtain both practical and emotional help from other people coping with similar problems. Ask at your doctor's surgery, Social Services department or library for details of local support groups such as a Parkinson's Disease Society branch, an Alzheimer's (a particular kind of dementia) support group or a general carers' group. You can also apply to the Social Services department (see your local phone book for their number) for an assessment of your wife's needs and your needs as carer. They will then be able to propose a package of services to meet your needs (see Chapter 4 for more information about these community care assessments).

Finally there are some very helpful booklets for carers of people suffering from confusion and dementia. We can particularly recommend a booklet called *Coping with Dementia: a Handbook for Carers* (see Appendix 2 for details) which is written in very carer-friendly language and is full of practical suggestions about what you can do to help your wife and yourself. Their summary of how to cope includes things like accepting your own feelings about what has happened, sharing the truth about the illness with others, looking after your own health and taking regular breaks.

My husband has had Parkinson's for the last six years but he has also developed some serious mental and behavioural problems and is not recognisable as the man I married. He keeps exposing himself and trying to touch any female who comes to the house. The result is that my friends are embarrassed to call and I am losing my friends as well as my husband. Please help!

This is an extremely difficult problem and we feel for you in trying to find a way of coping. The cause may be a side effect of the Parkinson's drugs, general mental deterioration which may or may not be due to Parkinson's, or frustration – or a combination of all three. If you have not already sought any help, we think that you should start by discussing the problem with your GP. Depending on his overall view of your husband's condition, he may suggest a referral to another specialist such as a psychiatrist or urologist.

Meanwhile there are some practical steps which you can take to make such behaviour less likely and less upsetting. First you can try to get him to wear clothing which is difficult to undo or take off such as dungarees (under a pullover they will look like ordinary trousers). Secondly you could try to screw up the courage to confide in your closest friends and see if they feel able to share the problem with you rather than hide away from it. It will help if you can reassure them that he really means no harm and is not fully responsible for his actions.

The other thing that will help is for you to have some days when you are not responsible for his care. You could try to arrange some day care through the Social Services department or hospital and, while he is away, try to get out and do something which you enjoy.

Outside the family

When my doctor sent me to see the consultant neurologist and Parkinson's was diagnosed, he explained quite well but

**seemed to imply that I was lucky it was Parkinson's. I don't
feel at all lucky – how could he think that?**

You have touched on an important topic which can lead to
mutual misunderstanding between doctors and their patients,
so it is helpful for us to have an opportunity to try and unravel
the issues. One of the most powerful influences on our satisfaction or dissatisfaction with things that happen to us is what we
are expecting, and that in turn depends in part on our previous
experiences. This is true whether we are talking about our
reactions to an evening out or to the news that we have a
medical condition like Parkinson's.

The worlds and experiences of medically-trained people like
neurologists and their non-medical patients are very different.
Without knowing what you thought the cause of your problem
might be, it's difficult to guess your first reaction to the diagnosis
but, if you did feel as shocked and dismayed as your question
suggests, you would not be unusual. There is no doubt that there
are lots of disadvantages to having Parkinson's including the
fact that, although treatment is available, there is as yet no cure.

A possible clue to your impression that your neurologist
thought you were lucky can be found in that last sentence.
Neurologists deal mainly with conditions for which, like Parkinson's, there is presently no cure but for many of the other
conditions there is no effective treatment either. In some
conditions (**not** Parkinson's) the life expectation after diagnosis
may be quite limited. So if you can imagine yourself in the
neurologist's place, knowing all that he knows, then you can
perhaps see why he feels much better about giving a diagnosis
for which he can offer some treatment and the hope of
improvement especially in the short and medium term.

However, understanding how such attitudes can arise does
not mean that they should be encouraged. If we want to
establish trust between people with Parkinson's and doctors so
that they can work well together over many years after
diagnosis, then doctors need guidance about how to give the
diagnosis and how to develop an attitude to Parkinson's which
is both honest and hopeful and which also acknowledges

people's fears and uncertainties. It is no help when you are grieving about breaking one leg to be told that you are lucky not to have broken two! When you can say such things to yourself, you know that you are beginning to come to terms with what has happened.

I work with a man who has Parkinson's. He is good at his job but seems very reserved and isolated. I don't want to intrude but wonder if I should encourage him to get more involved with other people at work?

Although people with Parkinson's are as diverse as anyone else in their personalities and attitudes, there are some aspects of the condition which make those who have it especially prone to isolation. If you are aware of these aspects, you will perhaps be able to explore them tactfully with your colleague and so discover whether his reserve is real and his isolation freely chosen. If he would like to be more sociable, it will be helpful for him to have your understanding and practical support.

The first thing to realise is that the rigidity of muscles in Parkinson's interferes with spontaneous movements and that it can lead to a 'mask-like' expression which makes smiling and showing interest more difficult. In these cases you might assume that someone is uninterested or bored when that is not the case at all.

On the other hand, people with Parkinson's sometimes withdraw from social contacts because they feel embarrassed by symptoms such as slowness, tremor or speech problems. If they can be helped to feel accepted and understood and given time to join in the conversation, they can become more confident again.

Finally, people with Parkinson's do tend to suffer from fatigue and, if they are doing a full-time job, this is especially likely. It may therefore be that your colleague has made a conscious decision to conserve his energies for work rather than socialising.

I manage to keep quite active in spite of having Parkinson's for more than five years. However my walking is rather

unsteady and passers-by sometimes stare or make comments as though I was drunk. It's very hurtful. How can we help people become more understanding?

We sympathise with your feelings of hurt about your experience, which is not that uncommon. You are right to focus on what we can do about it. Really it comes down to education – everything from public awareness campaigns and media coverage to information for individuals. The Parkinson's Disease Society (see Chapter 14 for more information) is constantly trying to devise ways of raising public awareness but there may be things you could do yourself. If you felt able to do so, you could stop and say that you have Parkinson's or perhaps hand over a small card (one available from the Parkinson's Disease Society is shown in Figure 8) which explains that you have a neurological condition which affects your walking and balance. Every little helps.

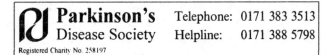

Parkinson's Telephone: 0171 383 3513
Disease Society Helpline: 0171 388 5798
Registered Charity No. 258197

I have Parkinson's disease

I may be slow to move or unsteady on my feet.
I may have difficulty speaking and writing clearly.
I can hear and understand you. Please allow time.

In case of emergency contact:

....

Figure 8: Information card produced by the Parkinson's Disease Society

6
Communication

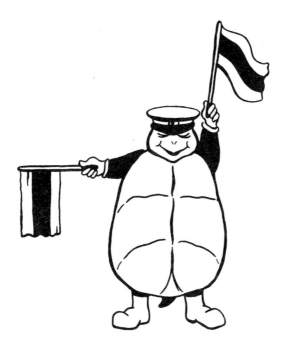

Introduction

The questions in this chapter are about **communication**, not just about **speech**, which is only one of the many ways we send and receive messages. Parkinson's can interfere with all the channels of communication and it can help to see these various aspects in relation to each other.

The Parkinson's Disease Society publish a leaflet called *Speech Therapy and your Speech/Language Therapist* (see Appendix 2 for details of how to obtain copies). This leaflet was prepared by the Speech Therapy Working Party and offers some general advice about how to recognise whether you have a communication difficulty and some suggestions to follow while trying to make that very important contact with your nearest speech and language therapist (see Chapter 4 for how to do this).

We cannot stress too strongly the major contribution of effective communication to a good quality of life and the importance, if you are experiencing difficulties, of obtaining early help and advice.

Getting your message across

I look in the mirror and find it difficult to recognise myself as my face seems so lacking in expression. Is there anything I can do to improve this?

Facial expression is a good example of an important kind of communication which is not speech. We all, perhaps without realising, take a lot of notice of the facial expressions around us. We may decide to give the boss a wide berth because he looks grumpy or pass several people in the street before we see someone who looks friendly enough to ask for directions.

There are several things you can do to help yourself and the first is to try and maintain a good posture – there is a question about this in Chapter 8. Perhaps surprisingly, our second suggestion entails looking in the mirror! Facial exercises, for example frowning and screwing up your eyes, then moving down your face to grins, yawns and smiles, can help to keep the muscles of your face more mobile and are best done in front of a mirror. Try saying a suitable word or phrase while doing these exercises – you could say 'lovely to see you' when you smile, for example, or 'I'm bored to tears' when you yawn. A special video and booklet called *Face to Face* has recently been produced by Iona Lister, a speech and language therapist with a particular interest in facial expression (see Appendix 2 for information on how to obtain copies). A local speech and language therapist or a physiotherapist will be able to suggest other, individualised, exercises for you to try.

The third thing you can do is to tell your relations and friends that lack of facial expression is one of the symptoms of Parkinson's and that they should assume that your face may be giving out inaccurate messages. We are afraid that you may have to repeat this message many times because our normal response to facial expression is deeply ingrained and we can be disconcerted and upset by, for example, the absence of smiles, even when we have been told that it is a common symptom of Parkinson's. Partners, relatives and friends may need to be helped to understand and make allowances for this feature, especially in the early days after diagnosis.

Are there particular exercises that I can do to help maintain my speech?

Yes there are, but which ones are most suitable will depend on how your speech is at the moment. If your current speech is good and you want to do everything possible to keep it that way, you could follow the suggestions in the leaflet *Speech Therapy and your Speech/Language Therapist* mentioned in the introduction to this chapter. Another important thing is to learn how to relax – an important skill for everyone but especially for people with Parkinson's. Good posture, as mentioned in the previous question, is part of this but you can also practise closing your eyes, breathing steadily and imagining a pleasant scene.

If you are already noticing some problems with your speech, you should contact your local Speech and Language Therapy Department as soon as possible (see Chapter 4 for more information about how to make contact with them). Do not be put off by mention of long waiting lists – ask at least to speak on the phone to a therapist with an interest in Parkinson's and explain your concerns. If talking on the phone is difficult, ask a family member or a friend to make the call for you.

I find that my voice is very quiet, almost a whisper. People –

even my family – find it difficult to hear me. Can you suggest anything to help?

A weak or quiet voice is not uncommon and we would recommend that you seek an assessment from a speech and language therapist who will be able to suggest exercises tailored to your particular needs. Meanwhile, here are a few suggestions – you probably won't be able to follow them all the time, but keep trying and you will perhaps find things a little easier.

- Try to keep your sentences short and precise.
- Think first what you want to say, then say it as simply as possible.
- Enunciate (use your tongue, lips and jaw in a somewhat exaggerated way) very clearly.
- Imagine that the room in which you are speaking is bigger than it really is.

The problem of a quiet voice may be made worse if older family members have some loss of hearing. If this is suspected, do encourage them to seek help too.

I have many friends who live some distance away so I rely on the telephone. However I find that the combined effect of my low voice and tremor are reducing my pleasure in these calls. Are there special phones which would help?

Yes. There are phones which you can use without holding the receiver, so helping to avoid problems from your tremor, and phones with amplifiers which will make your voice louder. Many phones now have memories, so you can store your most frequently used numbers and retrieve them by pushing just one or two buttons.

British Telecom has a special department to meet the needs of customers who have difficulties using the phone, and publishes a free guide called the *BT Guide for Elderly or Disabled People* showing the equipment and services available. This can be obtained from their local sales offices, or you can telephone BT and they will send you a copy (see Appendix 2 for details). Other makes of telephone may also have the same features and it might be worth checking to see if *Which?* magazine has a recent report on the best buys (your local library will probably have reference copies).

My father's speech has become very hurried, so much so that the words run into each other and are sometimes incomprehensible. What could be done to help him slow down?

Though not a very common problem, this does sometimes happen and it is very frustrating for the person concerned and for their relatives and friends. Try to get in touch with a speech and language therapist (see Chapter 4 for information about how to make contact) so that all aspects of your father's speech can be assessed. Encourage him to breathe deeply and steadily, to use short sentences and to vary the tone and volume of his voice as much as possible. The speech and language therapist will be able to suggest some exercises especially suited to his needs.

The thing I find really frustrating about my Parkinson's is the way my whole way of behaving and speaking is inhibited and slowed down. Sometimes I am longing to add my comments to a conversation but I can't get started. Any suggestions?

You have drawn attention to some very important matters. We convey a lot about what we are and how we feel by the way we use our bodies. Actors make conscious use of this method of communication but the rest of us do it because we cannot help ourselves. It is called body language (for obvious reasons) and, as with loss of facial expression, relatives and friends can help to minimise the impact which it has on relationships and communication by being aware of what is happening.

It would almost certainly be worth checking with your doctor to see if your Parkinson's medication could be changed in any way to give you more freedom of movement, though this is unlikely to remove the problem entirely. Medication which improves your general condition may help your speech but will not necessarily do so. You should therefore contact a speech and language therapist at your local hospital or health centre for more detailed advice (see Chapter 4 for information on how to make contact with them).

One tip for getting started is to breathe out through pursed lips while trying to imagine your listener's face sucking a lemon! You could also ask your friends and family to allow time for you to join in. Perhaps you could devise some sign which means 'leave a space for me'. Leaning forward in your seat, moving your head or touching someone's hand are all possible methods.

Your relatives and friends also need to be discouraged from speaking for you or finishing your sentences for you. Even those of us who ought to know better sometimes break these important rules.

Although he has had speech therapy in the past, my 55-year-old husband's speech is now quite poor and I think that we need an alternative method of communication. He is mentally alert but his hands are quite shaky so writing is not really possible. What choices do we have?

Your first and most important choice is to get in touch with your speech and language therapist again and see if she agrees with your assessment of the situation. If she does, she will be able to help you consider which of a wide range of communication aids will best suit your husband's needs. These can range from alphabet boards and very individual sets of signals, to relatively small and simple machines such as Lightwriters and Canon Communicators (see Appendix 1 for details of suppliers), to complex ones like computers. The most complex and expensive are not necessarily the best in every situation so it is very important to discuss the situation with an expert first. An advantage of the simpler systems such as cards or Lightwriters is that they are portable and so can be taken into less familiar situations, for example day centres or hospitals, where communication problems can be especially distressing. An advantage of the more complex (and expensive) systems, like computers, is that they may open up new interests for your husband if he has the patience and the will to learn how to use them. You will find more about this in the section on *Leisure* in the next chapter.

7
Work and leisure

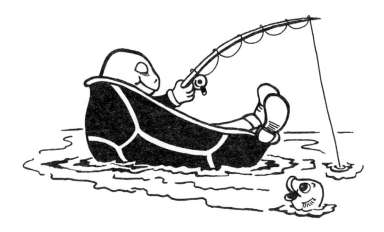

Introduction

For people still in full-time work, the onset of a permanent condition like Parkinson's can create considerable anxieties and uncertainties. In a climate of economic recession, such anxieties are exacerbated. Those who have decided to give up work or who have already retired face similar concerns about their capacity to go on doing the things which they enjoy – the things which reflect their personalities and help to make life worthwhile. This questions in this chapter are about these very important aspects of life and, like the questions in all the other chapters, they underline the great diversity of people with Parkinson's and the need to find individual solutions.

Work

I am 44 and was diagnosed 18 months ago. I am an estate agent. For how long can I expect to continue working?

This sort of question is always difficult to answer because Parkinson's varies so much from one person to another. And as you don't say how well you are at the moment, it is especially difficult to give you a clear answer. With effective medication people with Parkinson's can often continue working for many years. The introduction of apomorphine (which acts very quickly) means that, in people whom it suits, there is now even more chance of staying in employment. (See Chapter 3 for more information about apomorphine.)

It is easier to carry on working in some kinds of employment than others, especially in those which do not require great physical stamina or fast reaction times. Sometimes people with Parkinson's take early retirement, not because they cannot manage the job, but because they eventually find that the stress of work is interfering with their overall quality of life. The point at which a reduction in stress and more time for other activities outweighs the various advantages of remaining at work will be different for each person.

I work as a teacher in a large inner city school. It's interesting and challenging work but also stressful. Should I consider early retirement?

There is no 'should' involved here. Everything depends on how you feel, what your quality of life is while at work and whether, in order to keep working, you have to give up lots of the other activities which make life worthwhile.

Retiring from work is one of life's major turning points and should not be rushed into without balancing all the pros and cons. In this sense, you should certainly consider carefully before making such an important decision. Do not make a big decision like this if you are currently feeling depressed or shocked, for example because you have just been given the diagnosis. You should also be sure to give any new Parkinson's treatment adequate time to have an effect before making such decisions.

The financial implications of early retirement are often an important part of the equation (there is a question about this in Chapter 11) and it is vital that you obtain some good advice from a competent person. Often a personnel officer or a professional association or trade union is able to offer such advice, but, if not, you could approach the Welfare and Benefits Adviser at the Parkinson's Disease Society (address in Appendix 1).

Should I tell the people at work that I have Parkinson's? The treatment is working well but I know that there are some tell-tale signs and that I am slower than I used to be.

There is no answer to this question which is right for everyone, though we believe that the balance of advantage usually lies in telling the most important people such as your closest colleague and your immediate manager. If you are aware of 'tell-tale signs', the chances are that your colleagues at work have seen them too and are drawing their own conclusions. Their interpretations may be quite wrong and less complimentary than the truth! As we mentioned in Chapter 2, stress can make the symptoms of Parkinson's worse and, once you stop having to cover up, you may actually be able to do your job better.

However there will be circumstances, especially in a recession, when all jobs are at risk. Only you can know whether this risk is sufficiently grave in your own work situation to outweigh these arguments. We discuss these issues further in the answer to the next question.

What effects might my diagnosis have on my job security?

As we suggested at the end of the previous answer, much

depends on the kind of work you do and the general level of job security in your firm or employment sector. Obviously any kind of long-term illness can have an effect on job security. If your Parkinson's seems likely to have an early impact on your ability to do your present job, you should discuss this with your doctor to see if the treatment could be improved in any way. When you understand the medical situation fully, you should sit down and discuss the situation with someone who will help you to think through your options. You will find suggestions about whom this 'someone' might be in the answer to the next question. There is also a question further on in this chapter about how to obtain information on alternative jobs and retraining, and questions in Chapter 11 about the financial aspects.

What action should I take if I have problems in coping with my work or if my employer is not very understanding?

There are really two questions here. The first is about coping with work. It would be helpful to begin by clarifying in your own mind what the problems are. Then you need to talk things over with a good listener, preferably someone who knows about Parkinson's. You may know someone suitable already but, if not, you could contact the Parkinson's Disease Society (see Appendix 1 for the address and telephone number). They have a counsellor and a special telephone Helpline and will also know whether there is a local branch with a welfare visitor with whom you could discuss things. Once you have done this initial thinking, you will be able to identify other sources of advice and information such as your doctor, employer and employment disability services.

The second question relates to what you should do if your employer is not very understanding. The first actions would be those just described but you would need to add some consideration of the ways in which he or she is unhelpful and the chances of change if the situation was properly explained. The variable symptoms of Parkinson's can cause misunderstandings if the person concerned has not come across it before. If your conclusion is that your employer's attitude cannot be improved, then the balance would tip in favour of trying to find alternative employment or considering early retirement.

My husband is a qualified accountant but is unable to drive so is off work. Is there any way he could be helped to work from home?

Working from home is no longer uncommon - indeed, some people suggest that it is where nearly everyone will be working in the fairly near future. It can be particularly feasible for professional people who do not require lots of expensive equipment. Home computers which can be linked to those in the office offer many new possibilities of work from home. Your husband should first talk to his current firm to explore what options they can offer.

If they cannot offer home work, he could approach the Placing, Assessment and Counselling Team (PACT) at his local Jobcentre (listed under 'Employment Service' in the phone book). PACT has disability employment advisers who can offer a range of services to people with disabilities. It can help to be registered with the Employment Service as disabled and this can be arranged through these advisers. (We understand that accepting the label 'disabled' can be a difficult step to take but, if your husband can get over this hurdle, he will gain access to many sources of help.) To qualify for registration you have to be 'a person who, on account of injury, disease or congenital deformity is substantially handicapped in obtaining or keeping employment, or in undertaking work on his own account of a kind which ... would be suited to his age, experience and qualification'. The disability must be likely to last at least 12 months and the person concerned must be either in, or actively looking for work and have some prospect of getting it. Among the services available to people so registered are free permanent loan of equipment which helps to obtain or keep employment and help with fares to work where driving or public transport is inappropriate.

If your husband is thinking seriously of working from home, it will be worth doing some research into the possibilities and pitfalls. Any unemployed person can apply for help to set up their own small business through the Business Start-up Scheme run by the Training and Enterprise Councils (TECs) or in

Scotland by the Local Enterprise Companies (LECs). Any Jobcentre will have more details. There is also an association called the Telecottage Association (see Appendix 1 for their telephone number) which provides information and a support network for people working from home.

The other issue raised by your question is whether you have explored all the options for helping him to get to work. You will find more about this in Chapter 10 on *Mobility*.

Is specialised advice available about possible alternative jobs and retraining?

Yes. As mentioned in the previous answer, your local Jobcentre has a disability employment adviser who has special responsibility for helping people with a disability to find appropriate work and this includes retraining if necessary. Employment policy is in a state of constant flux and the criteria for admission to the various training schemes are detailed and complex so it is best to discuss your personal requirements with the adviser.

There are also private careers consultants who offer individualised advice although, of course, there is a charge for their services. To locate them, look in your local Yellow Pages under Careers Advice or Personnel Consultants.

Alternatively you could approach the Welfare and Benefits Adviser at the Parkinson's Disease Society (details in Chapter 14 and address in Appendix 1).

Leisure

My Parkinson's came on very slowly and has only recently been recognised. Meanwhile I seem to have given up lots of my old interests. Should I try to pick them up again now I'm receiving treatment?

Yes, definitely. We cannot emphasise too strongly the importance of keeping active and living as normal a life as possible. Your experience is not unusual when the symptoms come on very gradually, and it is a good sign that you are now thinking of picking up some of your old interests. Try one or two for a start, especially those you enjoyed most or which kept you in touch with friends, and see how things go.

My husband has always been interested in sport – as a player rather than a watcher. Are there any sports which seem particularly suitable for people with Parkinson's?

We know of people with Parkinson's who play almost every kind of sport, so there is sure to be something suitable for your husband. Energetic team games may pose some problems but tennis, squash, badminton, bowls, swimming, walking and snooker are just a few among many other possibilities. There is a British Sports Association for the Disabled (see Appendix 1 for the address) which he could contact if he has difficulty finding suitable local facilities, although many sports centres now make special provision for people with disabilities.

Alex Flinder won the Parkinson's Disease Society's first 'Mali Jenkins Welfare Essay Prize' for his report entitled *Bowls for the Parkinsonian* which is available from the Public Relations Department at the London office (address in Appendix 1).

One friend has told me that I will have to give up the active things I enjoy doing (which are dancing, walking, cycling and gardening) now that I have Parkinson's. Another friend disagreed, and said that it would be much better for me to keep on with them. Who's right?

There is no need for you to give up your activities because of your Parkinson's. Almost any form of exercise which you enjoy and which you can carry on safely and without undue fatigue is beneficial. The benefit comes in lots of different ways: physically in keeping your body fit and your joints and muscles in good condition; emotionally through the enjoyment and the sense of achievement; and socially because you get out and meet people and have things to think and talk about other than your Parkinson's. If you have any doubts about your chosen form of exercise, check with your doctor first.

The special advantages of music were discussed in the

question about music therapy in Chapter 3. Gardening is dealt with in the next question.

Gardening has been one of the passions in my life but the physical effort involved is beginning to detract from my enjoyment. Is there some way I can make things easier?

We sympathise – gardening is a major source of exercise, fresh air, creativity and enjoyment for millions of people and it is important to retain this interest for as long as possible. Luckily you are not the first person to feel this way and there is a Gardening for the Disabled Trust and another organisation called Horticultural Therapy, both with their own newsletters, which provide advice and practical help for gardeners with disabilities (see Appendix 1 for the addresses).

Other general information sources such as DIAL (Disablement Information Advice Lines) and the Disabled Living Foundation are also likely to have information about aids and equipment for gardeners. There is also an invaluable paperback full of good advice and information about equipment, seeds, manufacturers and relevant organisations. Called *Grow It Yourself* (details in Appendix 2), it will answer many of your questions and encourage you to continue cultivating your passion!

My wife, who has Parkinson's, and I have moved around the country a lot and have many old friends we would like to visit. However I am also somewhat disabled with arthritis and cannot drive any more. Is there anywhere we could get help in planning journeys to accommodate our combined disabilities?

Yes. There is an organisation called Tripscope (details in Appendix 1) which specialises in helping to plan travel for people with disabilities. If you are travelling by rail, the various rail businesses have a Rail Unit for Disabled Passengers and you can telephone their switchboard for assistance (the phone number is in Appendix 1). If you need an escort, you can usually get assistance from the St John's Ambulance Brigade or the British Red Cross and sometimes from local service organisations such as Rotary, Round Table, Lions or Soroptimists.

Would it be unwise to try to travel by air to Canada on my own? I am still active but carrying cases would be a strain.

Many people with Parkinson's enjoy international travel and there is no obvious reason why you should not go to Canada on your own. It will be sensible to choose a schedule which is not too demanding and which allows you to rest after the journey. If your only health problem is Parkinson's and the only foreseeable problem is coping with the luggage, then travelling by air is one of the safest and easiest means of travel. Airlines are particularly good about looking after passengers who need extra help, especially if you notify them beforehand. Check with your doctor anyway, just in case he or she has any special advice to offer.

Make sure that you have a good supply of your medicines with you and also a letter from your doctor stating clearly what medicines and doses are prescribed. This will be useful for your hosts if, by chance, you are unwell or need extra supplies and will help avoid any possible problems at customs, etc. We think it is a good idea to divide your medicines into two separate packages and store them in different bags so that if one bag goes missing, you still have an alternative supply. The Department of Health produce a very useful leaflet called the *Traveller's Guide to Health* (see Appendix 2 for how to obtain a copy). You should also make sure that you have adequate insurance cover for your holiday and that you have given full information on the application form about your Parkinson's and any other permanent medical condition (this is what insurance companies call 'pre-existing conditions'). Bon voyage!

My husband has always enjoyed writing – letters, diaries, poems, etc – and is very frustrated by how bad his handwriting has become. What can you suggest to help him maintain his interest in writing?

Deteriorating handwriting is a great source of frustration to many people with Parkinson's even if they do not also share your husband's literary interests. This handwriting problem is fairly easily resolved nowadays as long as your husband is willing and able to consider using a personal computer, word processor or electronic typewriter. The keyboards require less effort than old-fashioned manual typewriters and computers and word processors allow the written material to be corrected, amended and re-arranged any number of times before it is printed.

Try to get some good advice before you buy as there are so many competing models and packages on the market. *Which?* magazine has tested home computers and printers (your library will have back copies) and there is also a computer advice centre in Warwick called the Computablity Centre (see Appendix 1 for the address). We know of several people with Parkinson's whose lives have been transformed by access to a personal computer. (Please see Chapter 11 on *Finance* for information about obtaining help with the cost of computers.)

If for some reason a computer or electronic typewriter is not acceptable, then an even simpler option is a thick or padded pen or pencil, which can help improve grip and control. Weighted pens or wrist bands help some people and Dycem mats (which are made of washable, slightly sticky plastic) can stop the paper from sliding around. Your local occupational therapist (see Chapter 4 for how to make contact) will be able to offer advice on all these options and is also likely to have some suggestions about how the legibility of handwriting can be improved.

If a computer is the chosen solution and your husband needs training in how to use it, then he should approach your local further education college which is likely to have a range of courses in computing. We even know of people with Parkinson's who have been provided with home tutors. YAPP&RS, the section of the Parkinson's Disease Society for younger people with Parkinson's, has an active group of members interested in computers and is able to offer help, advice and encouragement. (See Chapter 14 for more details about YAPP&RS.)

One last suggestion – your husband may want to extend his interest in writing by joining a writers' group or class. There are many different kinds of opportunities, ranging from local further education courses to weekend residential courses to groups such as Writers' Own Publications (see Appendix 1 for the address) which help aspiring writers to get their work published.

**Reading has been a source of pleasure throughout my life but
is now becoming quite difficult due to a combination of
Parkinson's tremor and failing eyesight. Are there any aids
or organisations which might help?**

In answering this question we will assume that you have sought
medical advice about both the tremor and your eyesight. When
you are on the best possible treatment, there are several other
things you can do to help preserve this invaluable hobby. You
will find details of all the organisations mentioned below in
Appendix 1.

Firstly there are book stands which will help to hold the book
steady (ask your occupational therapist or contact the Disabled
Living Foundation, a local Disabled Living Centre or one of the
Keep Able shops to see what is available). Next, there are large
print books (Ulverscroft and Chivers are two of the largest
publishers) and books on cassette available in bookshops and in
most public libraries. Talking books are also available from the
National Listening Library (this library is available to all people
with disabilities, not just those with impaired vision). There are
also some newspapers on cassette available from the Talking
Newspapers Association UK. Lastly, if there are particular
papers, books or documents which you wish to read, large
public libraries often have special machines which can magnify
text or turn it into spoken words. You usually have to make a
booking for these machines.

**We love going to the theatre and concerts but my husband's
Parkinson's, which causes quite a lot of tremor and involuntary movements, is beginning to make this difficult. Do you
have any ideas to help?**

Our advice would be to contact the management of any cinema,
theatre or concert hall you want to attend and explain the
situation. Managements have begun to be much more aware of
the requirements of people with special needs but, to date, they
seem to have mainly considered the needs of people in wheelchairs and those with hearing difficulties. For your particular
problem, there may be some seats which would be especially

suitable or you may find that matinée performances are less crowded and so less likely to cause problems of distraction to others and embarrassment to your husband. London has an information service called Artsline and it would be worth checking with your nearest DIAL (Disablement Information Advice Lines – contact DIAL UK at the address in Appendix 1 for details of your local DIAL) or local authority information service whether there is anything similar in your area.

If you feel that you would like to campaign for improved access to public places for people with disablities, you may find that you have a local Access group doing just that.

I am a crossword and board game fanatic but am finding it increasingly difficult to cope with the fine hand movements required. How can I keep up my interest?

The various sources of aids mentioned in previous answers in this chapter, particularly the Disabled Living Foundation and the Disabled Living Centres, will have some games which are easier to manage. However, the best source of such games is now the home computer for which you can obtain crosswords, chess, bridge and many other traditional games as well as a vast array of modern computer games. There are many computer magazines on sale and in libraries which will have articles and advertisements about games programs.

If your fine hand movements remain a problem, you can explore the possibility of having a fingerguard fitted to your keyboard (check with the Computability Centre – the address is in Appendix 1) or try using a mouse rather than the keyboard.

Now that I have retired, I would like to fill some of the gaps in my formal education and general knowledge. What options do I have?

A huge number. Apart from colleges of further and higher education which are making special efforts to make their courses accessible to non-traditional students, there is also the Open University and the University of the Third Age (see Appendix 1 for addresses). All these organisations offer a wide range of courses and methods of learning, and cover academic subjects, current affairs, art, music, languages and much, much more.

My husband and I love visiting stately homes, old houses, gardens and so on, but sometimes they turn out to be unsuitable for his wheelchair and we end up being very disappointed. Is there some way of finding out whether a place is suitable in advance?

You can, of course, telephone most places in advance and it is certainly worth doing this if you are planning to travel a considerable distance. For general planning of outings and to cut down on telephone calls there are several useful publications.

For example, the *National Trust Handbook* gives information about the suitability of its properties for people in wheelchairs and also issues a separate guide to properties which are especially suitable. Some National Trust properties have motorised buggies available for people with mobility problems, and all give free admission to someone escorting a disabled person. Three other books giving details of wheelchair access are *Places That Care* by Michael Yarrow, the *National Gardens Scheme Handbook*, and *Historic Houses, Castles and Gardens* which includes 'over 1300 historic properties from cottages to castles'. Details of all these publications are in Appendix 2.

Other sources of information are RADAR (the Royal Association for Disability and Rehabilitation - their address is in Appendix 1) or, for ideas about places quite near to your home, try contacting some of the local groups for people with disabilities.

8
Managing at home

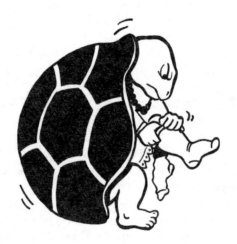

Introduction

With appropriate medication, adequate exercise and a healthy lifestyle, many people with Parkinson's have few difficulties in managing everyday tasks around the home. However, from the beginning quite a few have other medical conditions as well as Parkinson's, and so may meet additional problems. Others find that, as the years pass, things that were easy become more troublesome. Hardly anyone will have all the difficulties mentioned in this chapter so you need to find the questions which apply to you or to your partner, family member or friend.

There is a balance for everyone between independence and the selective use of equipment or new ways of approaching tasks – you may need to experiment to find out what is right for you. A new tool or technique can mean a real extension of independence for many people.

The Parkinson's Disease Society publishes a very useful booklet called *Living with Parkinson's Disease* (see Appendix 2 for further details). It has sections by a physiotherapist and an occupational therapist containing detailed diagrams, dos and don'ts, and lots of practical suggestions.

Mobility and safety

Getting up out of a chair is a real problem - have you any advice that will help?

Our first advice is to make sure that your regular chair is the right height (not too low), is stable and has arms on which you can push as you rise. Sometimes you may be able to adapt your present chair or you may want to buy a new one. Either way get some advice from your local occupational therapist or Social Services department. Once you are sure that your chair is suitable, try the following sequence of actions.

1. Move to the edge of the chair.
2. Place your feet on the floor, well under you.
3. Put your feet eight to 10 inches apart.
4. Put your hands on the arms of the chair (or on the sides of the chair seat).
5. Now lean forwards as far as you can from your hips. **This is very important**.
6. Press down on your feet and push forward with your arms and stand up.

These suggestions come from *Living with Parkinson's Disease*, which we mentioned in the introduction to this chapter. The booklet goes on to suggest ways of getting up when the chair is at a table and how best someone else can help if this is necessary.

How important is good posture and what can I do to maintain it?

Good posture is very important as it can have an influence on many of the other things you want to do, such as walking, balancing and talking. There seems to be a natural tendency for people to become a bit stooped or round-shouldered as they get older and this tendency is exaggerated in Parkinson's.

You may be surprised to learn that posture can affect talking, but this is because stooping constricts the lungs and makes it more difficult to breathe properly. So improving your posture can help prevent or alleviate speech difficulties (see Chapter 6 for more about speech and communication).

The first step towards improving your posture is to be aware of it. You can do this by standing or sitting in front of a mirror, noting your posture and trying to correct any faults you see. Study your 'improved' posture and then allow yourself to relax back into your normal posture. You should be able to feel as well as see the difference.

Here are a couple of exercises which will help you improve your posture and 'stand tall'. For the first, stand with your back against a wall and with the backs of your heels touching it. Now try to stand up as straight as you can so that your shoulder blades and the back of your head also touch the wall (illustrated on the left of Figure 9).

For the second exercise, you should stand facing the wall and a few inches away from it. Put the palms of your hands against the wall and stretch up as high as you can, watching your hands all the time (illustrated on the right of Figure 9). When you have stretched up as far as you can, hold the position for a count of five, and then relax.

Encourage your closest relative or friend to remind you to keep a good posture and it should get easier though, perhaps, never easy.

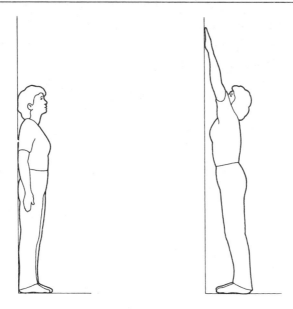

Figure 9: Posture exercises

I sometimes get stuck when approaching a doorway or narrow passage. Why should this happen and what can I do to solve the problem?

What you describe is a form of 'freezing', when you get stuck and cannot seem to get going again. No-one really knows why it sometimes happens in Parkinson's but it is thought to be related to incorrect balance or perhaps to an interruption in the messages from the brain to the muscles. It is one of the areas in which a whole range of 'try it yourself' solutions have grown up, as many people with Parkinson's have developed their own ways of getting themselves moving. All these solutions emphasise putting your heels to the ground first, to help you regain your balance and to keep it as you move. Once your heels are down, you can 'choose' from a whole range of options, including rocking from side to side, swivelling your head and shoulders to look at something alongside you, marching on the spot, swinging your leg backwards before trying to move forwards, stepping over imaginary lines, or even thinking 'provocative thoughts'!

What are the rules for turning round safely?

Living with Parkinson's Disease (see Appendix 2) offers the following straightforward advice: '... never swivel on one foot or cross your legs. Walk round in a semicircle, with your feet slightly apart. In other words, make the turn part of your walk. Always turn in a forward direction.'

We would add the following rules, especially for situations where there is a shortage of space.

1. Get your balance first before you start to turn.
2. Take your time – don't rush.
3. Do it in stages, for example make four quarter turns rather than one big one.

How can I improve my walking? I have a tendency to take very short steps or to shuffle.

Parkinson's can affect walking in lots of different ways and the effect varies from person to person and from one time to another. It's important to try to find the solution that is right for you because walking is an excellent form of exercise as well as a way of maintaining your independence and keeping up your interests and activities. Some of the following suggestions may help.

- Stop and take stock if you feel things are going wrong.
- Stand as straight as possible – leaning forward makes it more likely that you will either go too fast or get stuck.
- Put your heel down first and then your toe.
- Give yourself spoken instructions such as 'heel, heel' as you go along. (It is one of the strange aspects of Parkinson's that people who have it are sometimes able to do things when they put the actions into words, or when someone else gives them an instruction, even though they are unable to do them automatically.)

These suggestions are things which you can do for yourself, but there are physiotherapists with special experience in Parkinson's who could give you expert, individualised advice. To obtain this, you should ask your GP to refer you to a physiotherapist (see Chapter 4 for information about making contact).

I've always hated the idea of walking with a stick but now feel rather unsteady and am tempted to stay indoors. What walking aids are available?

We will assume that you have consulted your doctor and a physiotherapist so that your walking has been improved as much as possible. An ordinary walking stick with a non-slip ferrule (a rubber tip) does give some people quite a bit more confidence so we think you should probably try that first. Perhaps you could consider having an interesting or unusual stick or even a selection of different ones for different occasions! There are other walking aids such as tripod sticks, walking frames with and without wheels, folding frames, and trollies but they are more for use inside the house than outside. Walking-length umbrellas are **not** a good idea, as they are not secure enough to lean on.

If you do find you need anything more than a walking stick, it is really important to be properly assessed by a physiotherapist who understands about Parkinson's, as not all walking aids are suitable for people with Parkinson's.

Getting out and keeping up your interests is important so it is good that you are willing to revise your attitude towards something that may help. Confidence can also be boosted by having someone to accompany you when you go out. You may even want to consider 'wheels' some time, in which case you could look at the questions and answers in Chapter 10.

My wife gets really frustrated by her inability to turn over in bed and it's causing her to have bad nights. Can you suggest anything to help?

This is a little understood but very common symptom of Parkinson's – in one survey of members of the Parkinson's Disease Society, more than 60% reported this problem. Although there is unlikely to be a complete solution for her problem, there are several things which can help. We assume that your wife has checked her current medication with her doctor to ensure that it is at its best.

Having checked the medication, next check the bed! It is often easier to turn over on a firm mattress (if it is too soft, you could try putting a board underneath it). Some people find silky sheets useful, as they allow easier movement (see Appendix 1 under 'Silky sheets suppliers' for a source for these), or your wife could try wearing silky nightwear. Bedsocks may also make it easier to get a grip and so help turning over. *Living with Parkinson's Disease* (see Appendix 2 for details) illustrates two useful techniques for turning over in bed, one which your wife could try on her own and another which shows how you could help her if necessary.

Finally, if none of these proposals provides enough help, and if you can afford to spend some money to overcome the problem, there is a special 'Technabed' mattress which has been developed to solve this problem (see Appendix 1 for the supplier's name and address). Although not cheap, it is much less expensive than special beds with the same purpose. It can be used on an ordinary single or double bed and can be operated by the person with Parkinson's or the carer.

I live alone and getting out of bed (I have to, several times a night) is really difficult. Is there an aid which would help?

As we do not have enough information to consider whether your need to get out of bed so often could be tackled, we will answer the main gist of your question about how to help you get yourself out of bed.

Depending on the exact nature of your difficulty, the answer may be some techniques for getting yourself, by easy stages, into the right position. Once again we would suggest having a look at *Living with Parkinson's Disease* (see Appendix 2 for details) where several different methods are described and illustrated. Alternatively an aid like a bed pull which lies on top of the covers or a special frame by the side of the bed might be helpful. If your main difficulty is getting into a sitting position, you could consider an electrically operated bed, mattress or part-mattress. To determine which option is best for you, you need someone to come and assess you in your home so you should contact your local Social Services department or ask your doctor to refer you to an occupational therapist.

While at the doctor's, you might also discuss your need to get up so often during the night as there might be room for improvement there.

How can I reduce the risks of falling in the house?

In two ways. Firstly you can organise your home so that it is free from potential hazards such as slippery, polished floors, loose rugs and mats, trailing electric cables, and general clutter left on the floor. It will also help if you arrange your furniture to make moving around the house as easy as possible (for example, make sure that you don't have to avoid the coffee table every time you walk from your sitting room to the kitchen to get a cup of tea). Keep an eye open for pets - an affectionate cat or over-enthusiastic dog could also create hazards.

Secondly, you need to make sure that you are walking, turning round and getting out of your chair and so on as safely as possible (we have covered these topics in answers to earlier questions in this chapter). A special word of warning against reaching out for furniture to support yourself when moving around the house. Doing this could make falls more likely.

Although it is easy for us to say 'don't rush', we know that it is difficult to break the habits of a lifetime. However do **try** not to and, if there are particular occasions which tempt you to rush, such as the telephone ringing, consider placing a phone next to your usual chair, having some extra phones installed or switching to a cordless phone.

I have always enjoyed being a housewife and making my home attractive. Now people keep telling me to make it safe and I'm afraid it won't look like a home any more - and then I'll lose interest.

There is an important balancing act to be done here and we sympathise with your feelings about wanting to keep your home feeling like home. However with good advice from an occupational therapist and a little imagination and ingenuity from you, it ought to be possible to achieve something which is both reasonably safe and homelike.

We have to acknowledge that there can be no perfectly safe environment – and, if there were, its inhabitants would probably die of boredom! – so it's a question of compromise. It is also true that caring relatives and friends can become overprotective. You may need to sit down with them and talk about the freedoms you need and want to retain, and to acknowledge that the situation can be difficult for everyone involved.

I like to do my own cooking and cleaning but get tired easily and some days find such activities quite impossible. Do you have any tips which might help?

The first and most important tip is to time such chores for when you are at your best and to be prepared (with convenience foods and a conveniently blind eye for dust, etc) for days when you need more rest.

Of course we all use many labour-saving devices for preparing food and cleaning nowadays and you should make the maximum use of these. The kitchen especially needs to be organised in such a way that it is as safe and energy-efficient as possible. The expert in this field is the occupational therapist and, if you have not already requested a visit through either your GP or Social Services department, you should do so as soon as possible (see Chapter 4 for more information about making contact). She will also be able to recommend aids and appliances especially suited to your needs. Some are very simple such as non-slip mats to hold mixing bowls, padded handles, high stools and trollies. Others are more expensive and she may suggest a visit to your nearest Disabled Living Centre to try various models before deciding what to buy (see Appendix 1 for the Disabled Living Centres Council's address – they will give you details of your nearest centre).

Cooking can be a rewarding and enjoyable hobby as well as a practical necessity, so it is a good idea to try to maintain this interest. There is a useful and practical paperback called *Cook It Yourself* (see Appendix 2 for further details) which contains lots of easy recipes and short-cuts as well as ideas about useful

gadgets and kitchen arrangements. Each recipe has a nutri-
tional analysis so that you can check whether you are eating the
healthy diet recommended in Chapter 9.

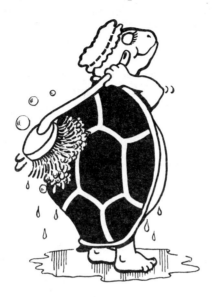

Personal care

**I pride myself on keeping clean and fresh but it's not easy
with stiff limbs and a tremor. There must be others, men and
women, in the same boat. How can we find out what aids are
available?**

There is a huge variety of aids available which range from simple
things like long-handled sponges to expensive specialised items
like lavatories that can wash and dry. You can get ideas about
some of the items which are available by looking at catalogues
such as those produced by Boots the Chemists (available from
their stores) or Chester-Care, or by arranging to visit your
nearest Disabled Living Centre or Keep Able shop (see Appendix 1 for addresses for the catalogues and the centres).

However, if you need anything other than very simple items,

you should ask your doctor to refer you to an occupational therapist who can see you in your own home (see Chapter 4 for more information about arranging this). Sometimes it is not just a question of the right aid but of how you tackle the task in question and an occupational therapist will be able to advise on both.

My mother, aged 75, loves to have a 'proper' bath but slipped recently in the bath and has lost confidence. I realise that we could have a shower fitted but is there any other solution to her problem?

One of the authors was once told that showers were all right for getting clean but if you wanted a deep, emotional experience, then a 'proper' bath was necessary! We think it is easy for professionals to underestimate the importance of baths as relaxation, especially for older people, so your question is an important one.

There are several lines of approach. You could try to help your mother feel more confident again by getting her to practise (with bare feet, of course, to prevent slipping) getting in and out of the bath while you are present. It can also help enormously if you, or someone else with whom she feels comfortable, can be around when she has a bath. There is also a wide range of appliances such as rails, mats and bath seats which might help or you could request help with bathing from your community nursing or home care service. The occupational therapist should be asked to call and assess the situation (see Chapter 4 for more information about how to make contact).

Another possibility is to see if there is a local nursing home which offers day care. Some of them have a variety of baths including 'walk-in' models, one of which might be especially suitable for your mother. Nearly all of these solutions might cost something depending on the arrangements in your local area and your mother's income. Using the nursing home would almost certainly be the most expensive unless the Social Services department agreed to provide it as part of a community care package (see Chapter 4 for more details).

I have been told that good dental hygiene is important and I

do try, but manipulating a toothbrush is now quite difficult. Is there anything which would help?

You are right about good dental hygiene being important – a healthy mouth and strong teeth contribute to good appearance and good diet. A padded handle on your toothbrush might help and some people find an electric toothbrush very useful. As with any other activities which you find difficult or tiring, you should choose a time of the day when your medication is working reasonably well. Mouthwashes may also be helpful. Be sure to keep in regular touch with your dentist (see Chapter 4 if finding a suitable one causes any difficulties).

It is also worth noting that any tasks such as toothbrushing, shaving, hairdrying and so on (all of which require controlled hand and arm movements) may be easier and less tiring if you support your elbows on a dressing table or other flat surface.

The monthly discomfort of my period is made worse by the practical problems of my Parkinson's. What advice can you offer?

First you need to talk with your doctor to ensure that both your Parkinson's and your periods are being managed as well as they can be. If you are lucky enough to attend one of the Parkinson's clinics which have a Nurse Specialist, then she would certainly be a good person to contact. An alternative would be the counsellor at the Parkinson's Disease Society National Office (see Appendix 1 for the address and phone number). A district nurse may also be able to offer help and advice.

You can feel very isolated with this kind of problem because the number of younger women with Parkinson's is relatively small, so you may like to consider joining the YAPP&RS (see Chapter 14 for more information). This is a special section of the Parkinson's Disease Society for younger people which enables you to exchange ideas with people who are likely to share some of your problems.

I have some gynaecological problems and I need to talk to someone about what can be done and how allowance can be made for the effects of my Parkinson's – I have both 'off'

times and fairly severe involuntary movements. Who could help me think things through?

As we said in the previous answer, the number of younger women with Parkinson's is relatively small so there are hardly any people around with the sort of combined expertise which you need. You are probably right to begin by finding someone with whom you feel comfortable enough to 'think things through'. This could be one of the YAPP&RS or a Parkinson's Nurse Specialist, the counsellor at the Parkinson's Disease Society National Office (address and phone number in Appendix 1) or someone you know locally. If you are under a neurologist, he or she may help you to discuss the options with a gynaecologist colleague so that you understand properly the pros and cons of various treatments. Attempts are being made through the Parkinson's Disease Society to get neurologists and gynaecologists together to discuss just these kinds of issues.

Dressing and undressing is such a hassle for people with Parkinson's especially if they live alone like me. What sorts of clothes are best and where can I find a good selection?

Yes, dressing and undressing can be difficult, and suitable clothes can make an important contribution to easing the problem. However, it is also important to choose a time when your tablets are working reasonably well and a place where you can be comfortable and warm so that you can take your time.

To return to the clothes: today's casual clothes with their elasticated waistbands and baggy tops can be ideal for people with dressing problems and have the added advantage that you can look like everyone else if you wish. Velcro, which is now used for fastenings on everything from waistbands to shoes, has been a great boon to people who have difficulty getting dressed.

The Parkinson's Disease Society publishes a leaflet on clothing which includes a list of stockists and there are also some special mail-order catalogue selections of clothes for people with dressing problems. A joint publication by the Disabled Living Foundation and the Parkinson's Disease Society called *Advice Notes for People with Parkinson's Disease* (see Appendix 2 for details) has an extensive section on clothing and a list of suppliers. It is important to have clothes that are easy to get on and off and which are both comfortable and attractive and *Yapmag* (the magazine of the YAPP&RS – see Chapter 14 for more information about both it and them) often has ideas on this subject. There is also some good general advice about dressing in *Living with Parkinson's Disease* (see Appendix 2 for more details of this booklet).

My mother, who has had Parkinson's for over 20 years, is beginning to have problems of urinary incontinence and is very distressed by it. What help is available?

Yes, this problem (which may or may not be related to her Parkinson's) is often distressing but there are things which can be done to help. First you should ask the doctor to examine your mother and identify the cause of the problem as there may be a specific treatment available. Secondly many Community Health Services (there is more information about these in Chapter 4) have specialist continence advisers so ask your mother's GP to refer her for a visit. They are skilled in advice about retraining the relevant muscles, in practical strategies to reduce the likelihood of accidents and in obtaining access to aids and/or laundry services if these become necessary. There is also a voluntary organisation called the Continence Foundation (address and phone number in Appendix 1) which offers information, advice and support to people coping with this problem. They run a confidential telephone Helpline so it is possible to discuss problems without giving names or feeling embarrassed.

9
Eating and diet

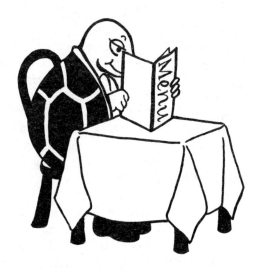

Introduction

Food, and the way we choose, prepare, present and control it, is a very important part of everyone's life. It can be especially important for people with long-term medical conditions and this is certainly true for people with Parkinson's. When we discussed attitudes in Chapter 5, we stressed the importance of helping yourself, of retaining interests and of feeling in control of your own life. A balanced approach to questions of eating and diet can contribute to all these aims.

Food and drink

What is the recommended diet for people with Parkinson's?

A normal, balanced diet with plenty of high-fibre foods such as wholemeal bread, wholegrain cereals, vegetables (particularly peas and beans), and fresh and dried fruit is recommended. It is also a good idea to drink plenty of fluids – about eight to 10 cups per day. The Health Education Authority produces attractive, free booklets about various aspects of healthy eating which can be ordered by post (see Appendix 1 for the address) or obtained from your local Centre for Health Promotion/Education if there is one in your area (see under Health in your local phone book for the address and telephone number). There is also a useful paperback called *Cook It Yourself* (details in Appendix 2) which offers some easy suggestions for balanced meals.

I prefer not to take medicines unless absolutely necessary but have quite a lot of trouble with constipation. How can I adjust my diet to help minimise this problem?

Follow the guidelines given in the previous question and be sure to have a breakfast containing wholegrain cereals. Pulses (peas, beans, lentils, etc) and dried fruit are particularly helpful. It is also important to take a reasonable amount of exercise if you can manage this. Do consult your doctor if the problems continue.

Can I eat chocolate whilst taking my Parkinson's medication?

Yes. For most people, chocolate creates no specific problems with Parkinson's medication although we have heard of some individuals who feel that it is unhelpful.

Is there anything in the idea that eating some kinds of beans can be beneficial?

As mentioned in the answers at the beginning of this chapter, beans are a good source of dietary fibre so in that sense they are helpful. However you may be alluding to some claims made about a particular variety called *vicia fabia* beans which have been promoted by a Mr Dan Beth-El from Israel. These beans are claimed to contain L-dopa (which is probably true though far less than in the normal tablets prescribed for Parkinson's) and an extra ingredient which makes the L-dopa work more effectively (which is unproven, though several studies are being started to test the claim). On present evidence, no one should alter their drugs without discussing any changes with their consultant or GP.

Is it true that foods containing protein can make my wife's Parkinson's worse?

This is an interesting question on a topic about which doctors and researchers are still divided. It is true that protein can interfere with the absorption of L-dopa by the brain and thus cause a dose of L-dopa taken with or after a protein-rich meal to be less effective. Severe restriction of daytime protein has been tried in people who have serious Parkinson's symptoms and, in some tests, they have shown a marked improvement in response to their L-dopa medication. However, not everyone is helped, the diet is rather unpalatable and therefore difficult for people to sustain, and there are some indications that marked reduction of protein and increase in carbohydrate (sugar, bread, pasta, etc) can lead to more involuntary movements. Another potential complication is that some recent research has suggested that people with Parkinson's, especially those with severe muscle rigidity, use up more energy than people of the same age and sex who do not have Parkinson's and that this may help to account for the excessive weight loss in some people. Restriction of protein intake would make it more difficult to treat such loss of weight.

In general, doctors and dietitians are not in favour of restrictive diets which take away one of life's main pleasures but, for people experiencing major difficulties, a low protein diet (or more simply just eating less protein at one meal) may be worth considering or trying for a while. **It should only be undertaken after discussion with the neurologist or other specialist and under the supervision of a dietitian** – the body needs a certain amount of protein to renew itself and to help it fight infection so restricting protein may precipitate other problems.

What is a normal amount of protein?

It is easier to say what is 'recommended' rather than what is 'normal' because some people in the richer countries tend to eat more protein than they need. The amount recommended depends on body weight and is about 0.9 grams per kg of body weight per day. This would mean that a person weighing 11 stones (70 kg) should eat about 60 grams (about 2 oz) of protein per day. However, for all the reasons given in the answer to the previous question, there are other considerations in people with Parkinson's and reduction or redistribution of protein should only be tried under medical and dietary supervision.

I like a drink (mostly beer) with my friends. Is this all right or will it interfere with my Parkinson's medication?

Alcohol taken in moderation will not interfere with your medication and, if it helps you continue with your normal way of life, it will probably do you good. Obviously everyone, with and without Parkinson's, should avoid excessive drinking.

I have heard that Vitamin B_6 should be avoided by people with Parkinson's. Is this correct?

This vitamin was a potential problem in the early days when L-dopa was not combined with a special inhibitor to prevent the L-dopa breaking down before it reached the brain. Excessive amounts of Vitamin B_6 made the problem worse. Now that almost everyone takes medication (such as Sinemet and Madopar) which contain an inhibitor, there is no problem. Excessive amounts are still best avoided and, if you feel a need for vitamin supplements, you should be able to find some which do not contain vitamin B_6. Quite a lot of research is taking place to investigate whether certain other vitamins, particularly C and E, might be helpful in slowing down the damage to dopamine-producing cells in the brain, but so far the results are inconclusive.

Is it true that brown bread contains manganese and that this is a possible cause of Parkinson's and so should be avoided?

It is true that manganese poisoning can cause symptoms similar to those of Parkinson's but this condition is found only in miners in manganese mines and is extremely rare. It is not true that brown bread should be avoided. There is no indication that the ordinary dietary intake of manganese from foods such as brown or wholemeal bread has any effect on Parkinson's. There is evidence that diets low in fibre are more likely to lead to problems with constipation, a common accompaniment to Parkinson's, so there are definite advantages in eating wholemeal bread.

Eating and swallowing

Eating was one of my mother's main pleasures. Now her tremor and stiffness make mealtimes slow and difficult and she hates to be helped.

Most of us would be very upset if we needed regular help with feeding, so your mother's wish to remain independent is entirely understandable. There are things which can help although they all require some tolerance of special arrangements and special equipment.

Smaller, more frequent meals of easily-managed foods will ease the problem of slowness and special plates to keep food warm can help too. Raising the plate so the distance from plate to mouth is reduced can help to minimise the effects of tremor, as can supporting the elbows on the table. There are many different designs of cutlery and crockery to improve grip and to reduce the likelihood of spillage. These include plate guards, two-handled cups and tumble-not mugs. There are also special eating systems such as the 'Neater Eater' which has a long arm with 'dampers' to reduce the effects of tremor. You can find these items and many more in catalogues such as those from Boots the Chemists (available from their stores), Chester-Care and Keep Able (see Appendix 1 for addresses), but the best way to get an assessment of the whole situation, and recommendations especially suitable for your mother, is to contact an occupational therapist through her doctor or Social Services department (see Chapter 4 for more information on how to make contact). The occupational therapist may suggest a visit to one of the Disabled Living Centres (see Appendix 1 for the Disabled Living Centres Council's address – they will give you details of your nearest centre).

My father has great difficulties in swallowing. What kind of diet should he have to ensure that he gets enough nourishment?

This is a distressing problem found in some people with long-standing Parkinson's. If your father has not been seen by a speech and language therapist to have this problem fully investigated, you should try to arrange this straight away through your GP (see Chapter 4 for more information about making contact). The speech and language therapist will be able to suggest some ways of coping with the problems and will also be able to put you in touch with a dietitian who can give specialist advice about adequate nutrition. Meanwhile here are some suggestions.

- **Avoid** mixed textures like liquid with bits such as watery mince and some soups; and flaky or dry foods such as nuts, hard toast and some biscuits.
- **Use** wholemeal bread rather than white bread which tends to form a solid mass and is harder to swallow.
- **Include** some protein-rich foods such as meat, fish, eggs, cheese and milk, and some energy-rich foods such as butter, margarine, cream, mayonnaise, sugar, glucose and honey.
- **Purée or thicken** foods to an even consistency. If you purée foods, try to do them separately so that they retain their own colour as it is important that food remains appetising. Possible thickeners are milk powder, instant potato powder, custard, wholemeal flour, beaten egg, yoghurt, cooked lentils and tinned pease pudding. You could also use a proprietary thickener like Carobel which is obtainable from a chemist.

Are there any other hints to help people with swallowing problems?

Yes there are, but we cannot stress too strongly the need to get expert, individualised advice from a speech and language therapist. The Parkinson's Disease Society publish a useful leaflet called *Speech Therapy and your Speech/Language Therapist* (see Appendix 2 for more details) which contains several suggestions. These stress the importance of good posture and taking enough time, and include hints such as lowering the chin towards the chest before swallowing, clearing the mouth and throat completely after each bite or spoonful, and sipping very cold fluids before or with meals.

10
Getting around on wheels

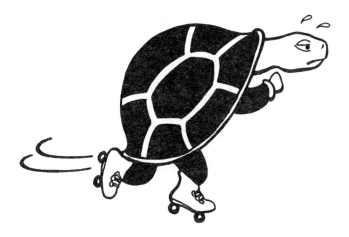

Introduction

This chapter is all about getting around on wheels - not, we hasten to add, the skates of our intrepid mascot, but the wheels on cars, pavement vehicles, scooters and wheelchairs. Although most people with Parkinson's do not use a wheelchair and some have never been car drivers, these are very important topics for those to whom they apply. Most people are car passengers from time to time so questions about easier entry to and exit from cars may be relevant to anyone with mobility problems.

Almost everyone recognises the difference which a car can make to their independence and mobility, but wheelchairs are too often seen not as a useful set of wheels but as a symbol of disability. While not in any way wishing to underestimate the distress attached to needing a wheelchair, we do want to encourage the minority of people with Parkinson's who do eventually need a wheelchair to see that using one can widen horizons which may have become very narrow.

For additional information and advice on any of these matters, you can contact the Welfare and Benefits Adviser at the Parkinson's Disease Society; the Disabled Living Foundation in London or regional Disabled Living Centres; or your local DIAL (Disabled Information Advice Line) group. If a telephone number for DIAL does not appear in your local phone book, then DIAL UK, which coordinates the local groups, will be able to provide further information. You will find addresses and telephone numbers for all these organisations in Appendix 1.

Getting around without a car

I'm not at all keen on the thought of a wheelchair but my children are urging me to consider having one. How can I discover which type is best for me?

First you need to discuss with your doctor and a physiotherapist whether you do need a wheelchair and, if so, whether for indoors or outdoors. If they and you agree that a wheelchair would help, you can be referred to the local NHS wheelchair centre where you will have an assessment to establish which type of wheelchair will be best for you. Not all types of wheelchair are available on the National Health Service but an objective assessment will help you to know what choices are available.

If you feel that you would like to borrow one first to gauge how you will feel, short-term loans can usually be arranged with your local British Red Cross Society, St John's Ambulance Brigade or Age Concern. Look in your local phone book for the numbers.

Since I gave up driving, I get out of the house much less and I really miss getting around to see old friends, go shopping, etc. I do get a taxi sometimes but it is rather expensive. What else is available?

It is not clear from your question whether your physical condition or finances would allow you to consider having a pavement vehicle of some kind. If so, read the answer to the next question. Otherwise, what is available depends on the area in which you live, but we will mention some of the likely alternatives. Many areas have a special Dial-A-Ride minibus service for people who have mobility problems. You first have to join the scheme – and sometimes there is a waiting list. Once accepted, you can ask the minibus to collect you from your own home and bring you back and the charge is very modest. Some areas have a system of taxi vouchers for people who are unable to take advantage of free or concessionary bus fares.

While thinking about taxis, it is worth saying – especially to those who used to run their own cars – that you can have a very large number of taxi journeys for what it costs to keep a car on the road. It can be a useful exercise to work out the amounts. If the cost of transport is a problem and you are under retirement age, check if you are eligible for the Mobility Component of the Disability Living Allowance (see the section on **Money and mobility** later in this chapter for more information about this).

For journeys outside your local area, there is an organisation called Tripscope (see Appendix 1 for the address) which can help you plan journeys and from which you can also obtain escorts if these are required. Other sources of escorts are the St John's Ambulance Brigade, the British Red Cross Society and local service organisations such as Rotary, Round Table, Lions and Soroptimists.

My walking has been poor for some time and I have an ordinary wheelchair which I can use around the house and which my friends can push when we go out. However I would like to be more independent and am wondering about a pavement vehicle. How do I go about finding out more?

There is a wide variety of pavement vehicles to suit differing individual needs and different outdoor conditions. As outdoor powered vehicles for control by the user are not available through the National Health Service, you will need to have funds to pay for your pavement vehicle. It is possible to buy electric wheelchairs as well as cars under the Motability hire purchase scheme (there is a question about Motability in the *Money and mobility* section later in this chapter).

First you need an assessment of the type of vehicle most suited to your needs. You can visit (by appointment) the Disabled Living Foundation's Equipment Centre in London or one of the Disabled Living Centres around the country (see Appendix 1 for addresses). The Banstead Mobility Centre also offers assessments for a modest charge, and a range of information leaflets about wheelchairs.

Most suppliers have showrooms or may even make home visits to demonstrate their models (but do not be pressurised into buying without independent advice and time to consider all the options). Some firms supply reconditioned second-hand vehicles and many specialist magazines and voluntary organisation newsletters carry advertisments for second-hand models.

Pavement vehicles, whether wheelchairs, scooters or buggies can make a major contribution to independence and quality of life, but they are not cheap, so be sure to try them out and get good advice before deciding to buy.

Cars and driving

I like to take my father out shopping or for a drive sometimes but getting him in and out of the car is becoming more difficult. Are there ways of easing this problem?

Yes, there are. Which one you choose depends on your father's needs, your particular type of car and how much you want to pay. There is a very simple swivel cushion made by AREMCO (see Appendix 1 for address) which you put on the passenger seat and which allows the legs to be swung round into the car much more easily. Less simple and more expensive but very effective is the adaptation or replacement of the whole passenger seat so that it can be turned to face the pavement and then be moved round to the front again once the passenger is seated (see Appendix 1 under 'Swivel car seats suppliers' for names and addresses of suppliers).

Is it true that I have to notify the DVLA about my Parkinson's?

Yes. Parkinson's is one of a number of medical conditions which can affect driving ability and which therefore have to be notified in writing to the DVLA (the Driver and Vehicle Licensing Agency – see Appendix 1 for the address). They will then send you a PK1 form (Application for a driving licence/Notification of driving licence holder's state of health) to fill in and return.

For information on what happens after you receive the form, read the answers to the following questions.

Could I lose my driving licence?

You could, but it is unlikely especially if you have only been diagnosed recently. The DVLA will study the information on your completed PK1 (the form mentioned in the answer to the previous question) and if satisfied that your driving ability is not a hazard to other road users will, in the majority of cases, issue a three year licence. At the end of three years, they will review your situation.

The DVLA wants to give drivers with a current or potential disability the best chance of keeping their licences but it is also responsible for public safety. It is helpful to know how the system works. For example, there are a series of questions on the reverse side of the notification form (PK1) to which you have to answer 'yes' or 'no'. If your answer to any of questions 2–11 is 'yes', you should send a covering letter in which you clarify your answer and explain why you still consider that you are fit to drive. If you do not do this, you may find that your licence is withdrawn unnecessarily.

It is also helpful to discuss your driving ability with your GP and specialist as the DVLA may contact them for their opinions.

If there is any disagreement between your doctors and yourself or if you have some concerns about your driving abilities, it would be worthwhile trying to arrange for an assessment at one of the specialised driving or mobility assessment centres (see Appendix 1 under 'Mobility Assessment Centres' for addresses). There is a question about these centres later in this section.

What does my GP know about my driving ability?

Your GP should know how your medical condition is affecting your use of your hands and legs, and how it could interfere with other faculties like vision which are essential for safe driving – though even for some of this he will need good and accurate information from you. Unless he or she has driven down the road behind you, it will not be possible to judge your general driving ability! The variability of Parkinson's itself and, in some people, the unpredictable nature of their response to medication, makes all these judgements more difficult than in some other conditions. That is why it is so important to discuss your driving with your doctor and to request a special driving assessment if there is any disagreement or uncertainty.

How do I arrange for a driving assessment?

You should contact your nearest driving assessment centre (see Appendix 1 under 'Mobility Assessment Centres' for addresses). These are specially staffed and equipped centres around the country which will test your driving capabilities (with adaptations if necessary) and write a report. This report will help you decide whether you want to go on driving and may be essential evidence if you do lose your licence and want to appeal against the DVLA decision (there is a question about making an appeal later in this section).

There is a charge for these assessments which varies between centres and with the type of assessment required, so it is important to ask for information on charges when you contact the centre. If you have difficulty meeting the charges, the Welfare and Benefits Adviser at the Parkinson's Disease Society (address in Appendix 1) may be able to help.

My driving ability is now rather variable, depending on how I am feeling and how well my tablets are working. I don't want to lose my licence but I don't want to be a danger to myself and others either. What shall I do?

We sympathise with your dilemma which will be shared by several other people with Parkinson's. You first need to talk to someone who understands about both Parkinson's symptoms and about driving assessments so we suggest that you contact the Welfare and Benefits Adviser at the Parkinson's Disease Society (address in Appendix 1). It should then be possible to decide whether to proceed with a full driving assessment at one of the centres described in the answer to the previous question.

My husband's licence has been withdrawn by the DVLA and he is devastated. We both feel that he is fit to drive – do we have any right of appeal?

Yes, your husband has the right to appeal and, to use it, he should write immediately to the DVLA (Driver and Vehicle Licensing Agency) giving notice of his intent to appeal. Even those who are unsure whether to appeal or not are advised to register their intent to do so as appeals have to be lodged quite soon after notification of the DVLA decision – within six months in England and Wales, and within one month in Scotland. The application to appeal can be withdrawn at any time prior to the hearing. All driving licence appeals are heard in the Magistrates' Court (or, in Scotland, in the Sheriffs' Court).

It is extremely difficult to succeed with an appeal unless you have some new evidence – from your doctor or from a driving assessment centre – which was not available at the time of your original application to the DVLA. We would strongly advise that your husband discusses the matter with someone who has special experience in such cases. Possible sources of such advice are your local DIAL (Disability Information Advice Line), your Citizens' Advice Bureau, and the Welfare and Benefits Adviser at the Parkinson's Disease Society. It is very important to be clear about your chance of succeeding with an appeal before going to the hearing because, apart from the distress that an unsuccessful appeal can cause, the DVLA normally seeks to recover its costs (which are likely to be several hundred pounds) if the Court upholds its original decision.

My husband does not want to tell his insurance company about his Parkinson's as he is afraid they will stop him driving. Could they do this?

The answer to this apparently simple question is 'no' and 'yes'. It is not the insurers but the DVLA (Driver and Vehicle Licensing Agency) which is able to decide whether your husband is fit to drive and so may have a driving licence. However, it is illegal to drive on public roads without at least third party insurance, so the insurance company does have some influence on whether a person is able to drive or not. Your husband **must** notify his insurance company that he has Parkinson's.

All insurance companies require their clients to tell them the full facts about any disabilities or serious illnesses they may have and about all adaptations made to their cars. Failure to do this will probably invalidate your husband's insurance. Not only could this present problems with any claim he might make in the future, it would also mean that he was driving illegally. The main problem your husband could face is increased premiums but these are not inevitable, and it is very important to shop around and get several quotations before making a final decision. It is also essential to read any potential policy thoroughly, including the small print. By doing this, your husband will be able to judge what he is getting for a particular premium. If your husband's present insurance company increases his premium **because of his Parkinson's**, it would be worth contacting some of the insurance brokers which special-ise in insuring disabled drivers. A list – *RADAR Mobility Factsheet 6* – with indications about the kind of cover on offer can be obtained from RADAR (Royal Association for Disability and Rehabilitation) at the address given in Appendix 1. We have recently heard of someone who used one of these specialist brokers and whose premium is now lower than it was before his diagnosis!

Money and mobility

Is there any financial support available to help people who have mobility problems?

Yes, though not everyone with mobility problems will be eligible. There is a Department of Social Security (DSS) benefit for this purpose which used to be called the Mobility Allowance. This was replaced in April 1992 by the Mobility Component of the Disability Living Allowance (DLA). Anyone who had the Mobility Allowance before April 1992 should have been automatically transferred to the DLA Mobility Component. Anyone under 65 (or under 66 if the disability began before the age of 65) applying since April 1992 is assessed against the disability rules. If they are 'unable or virtually unable to walk (with aids if used)', they qualify for the higher rate and if they are 'able to walk but need the guidance or supervision of another person most of the time when walking outdoors', they qualify for the lower rate.

Obviously there are specific rules and procedures which are difficult to spell out in detail here, so if you think that you may be eligible do telephone or write for a claim pack from the Benefits Agency (the organisation that handles social security payments for the DSS – it will be listed in your local phone book). Try also to discuss the matter with someone knowledgeable like your local DIAL (Disability Information Advice Line) group or the Welfare and Benefits Adviser or a branch welfare visitor at the Parkinson's Disease Society (addresses in Appendix 1). The variability of Parkinson's can create particular problems in establishing eligibility for this and other benefits so it is especially important to get advice from an experienced person. There are also review and appeal procedures which you can use if you disagree with the decision made by the adjudication officer or if your circumstances change. A leaflet – *RADAR Mobility Factsheet 8* – with useful and detailed information on all these matters can be obtained from RADAR (Royal Association for Disability and Rehabilitation) at the address given in Appendix 1.

It is important to establish whether you are eligible for one of the rates of the Mobility Component of DLA because, once granted, they can help you to get other benefits. The rate payable on this Mobility Component can also effect the level of other benefits such as Severe Disablement Allowance, Disability Working Allowance and Disability Premium. There is more information about benefits and other financial issues in Chapter 11 on *Finance*.

Wheelchairs, pavement vehicles, crutches and walking frames are exempt from VAT (Value Added Tax).

What special help is available for drivers?

Those drivers who are granted the higher rate of the Mobility Component (see the answer to the previous question) are eligible for exemption from vehicle excise duty (road tax) on one car. Technically, the vehicle is only exempt when it is being used 'solely by or for the purposes of the disabled person' but, unless there is flagrant abuse of the exemption, there is unlikely to be any trouble.

People receiving the higher rate of Mobility Component are also automatically eligible for an orange badge (which gives them important parking privileges) and for access to Motability schemes (there is a question about Motability later in this section). They also get relief from VAT (Value Added Tax) on adaptations which make their cars suitable for use by disabled people, and on the installation, repair and maintenance of these adaptations.

Do Mobility Component payments count as income for other purposes such as taxation or means-tested benefits?

No, they are not taxable and should not be taken into account as income for other benefits. Nor should any arrears count as capital for means-tested benefits for up to a year after they are paid.

What is Motability?

Motability is a special scheme, available to drivers who have the higher rate of Mobility Component, which helps them to hire, purchase and maintain their cars. It is administered through certain garages and involves handing over the benefit in exchange for certain services. For more information you should contact the head office of Motability (see Appendix 1 for the address).

11
Finance

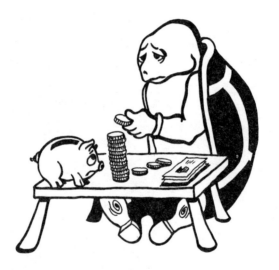

Introduction

People who have a long-term illness and/or who are elderly often have special needs for treatment, care or equipment. These special needs can significantly increase their living expenses and this is certainly the case for many people with Parkinson's. This chapter provides an outline of some of the main sources of financial support. Other general topics with a financial aspect such as mortgages, insurance policies and prescription charges are also included here, but the money side of motoring is discussed in Chapter 10, and the financial aspects of care outside the home are dealt with in Chapter 12.

This chapter covers a very complex area of knowledge with many detailed rules and allowances for special circumstances. Not only is it complex, it is also subject to change as the benefits system in this country is reviewed at frequent intervals. People who are in any doubt about their entitlement or who want to question their current levels of financial support will need to make further enquiries. Sources of help include the Benefits Agency (the organisation which handles social security payments for the Department of Social Security); the local Citizens' Advice Bureau; or your local authority's welfare rights adviser (all of these organisations should be listed in your local phone book).

You can also contact the Welfare and Benefits Adviser at the Parkinson's Disease Society (address in Appendix 1) or the welfare visitor, where available, at a local branch of the Parkinson's Disease Society. All of these people and organisations should also be able to provide information about the current levels of various benefits.

Benefits

I am 36, single and over the last few months have been either unemployed (I lost my job six months ago) or off sick (when control of my Parkinson's symptoms causes trouble). I am finding it increasingly difficult to manage financially – what help is available to me?

A combination of current shortages of employment opportunities and the fluctuating nature of your Parkinson's has placed you in a difficult position. You should certainly talk to your doctor about the chances of improving the control of your Parkinson's, and to a disability employment adviser at your local Jobcentre about employment and/or retraining possibilities (you will find more information about this in the section on *Work* in Chapter 7).

If you remain off sick or unemployed, you can apply for Income Support (a non-contributory means-tested benefit). If you are considered incapable of work you may be eligible for Incapacity Benefit (a new benefit which has replaced both Invalidity Benefit and Sickness Benefit, and is intended to provide for both short-term and long-term incapacity) and for Disability Living Allowance (discussed in the answer to the next question). At the time of writing, exact regulations for Incapacity Benefit had not been finalised, so we would suggest that you ask either the Welfare and Benefits Adviser at the Parkinson's Disease Society (address in Appendix 1) or someone at the Benefits Agency for further information.

If you return to work but at relatively low rates of pay you may be entitled to a new benefit called the Disability Working Allowance. There are both advantages and disadvantages vis-à-vis other entitlements to applying for the Disability Working Allowance, so you should be sure to talk to someone who can help you do this calculation. There should be a nominated person in each Social Security or Unemployment Benefit office who can give you information, or you could approach one of the organisations or people mentioned in the introduction to this chapter. You will find Social Security offices listed under 'Benefits Agency' in your local phone book, while Unemployment Benefits offices will be listed under 'Employment Service'.

What is the Disability Living Allowance and who can claim it?

The Disability Living Allowance (which replaced Attendance Allowance for people aged 65 and under) is paid to people who require personal care or supervision by day or night and/or to people who have considerable mobility problems. It has separate care (three levels) and mobility (two levels) components so people with a wide range of different needs may be eligible. Application forms can be obtained by ringing the Benefits Agency freephone number (listed in your local phone book) or from the Welfare and Benefits Adviser at the Parkinson's Disease Society (address in Appendix 1). It is important to obtain the support of your GP or other health professional as the application form contains a space for their comments.

Who is eligible for Severe Disablement Allowance?

People under pensionable age who have an insufficient contribution record to claim Incapacity Benefit (which has replaced both Invalidity Benefit and Sickness Benefit) and who can satisfy an 80% test of disablement are eligible for this benefit. The test is conducted by a medical examiner appointed by the Department of Social Security and we understand from the Welfare and Benefits Adviser at the Parkinson's Disease Society that people with Parkinson's who are unable to continue working generally succeed in their applications. The Severe Disablement Allowance counts as income for the calculation of all other benefits except Attendance Allowance and Disability Living Allowance.

My father has received the lower rate of Attendance Allowance for the past two years but now needs more supervision. Can he apply for the higher rate and how is the decision made?

Attendance Allowance is for people aged 65 and over who need a lot of care or supervision. If circumstances change he (or you on his behalf) can apply for a review at any time. Just write to the local Attendance Allowance office (the address will be on the letter granting his original allowance or can be obtained from your local Benefits Agency office) with an explanation of the change in circumstances. Your letter will be acknowledged and they will make various enquiries to establish whether or not he is entitled to the higher rate. These enquiries could include letters to your father and to his doctor or consultant and, in some cases, a special medical examination.

You are more likely to succeed with your claim if you get help and advice from someone with previous experience of such applications, such as welfare experts at national or branch levels of the Parkinson's Disease Society (address in Appendix 1). People applying for this benefit for the first time are also advised to obtain some expert help in completing the application form. The form is available from the Post Office, the Benefits Agency or the local Attendance Allowance office.

We applied for Attendance Allowance for my wife but were refused. Is it worth appealing?

Formal appeals are now much rarer than they were in the past and most disagreements get sorted out either by a re-application or, if the refusal came within the last three months, by a review. If you feel that you have a case, it is certainly worth pursuing the matter as many applications which fail the first time are granted on review. Please read the answer to the previous question and try to obtain some expert help in completing the form. It is easy with something variable like Parkinson's to give an unrealistically optimistic picture of the situation.

I do not live with my elderly mother-in-law but I share the task of caring for her with my sister-in-law. She gets Invalid Care Allowance – is it possible that I could be eligible too?

No, only one person can claim Invalid Care Allowance for a particular disabled person but, if you are spending a minimum of 35 hours per week looking after your mother-in-law, you can claim Home Responsibilities Protection for each full year spent caring. This can help to protect your own pension rights so it is worth applying.

Is there any help available with the cost of prescriptions for Parkinson's drugs?

The disappointing answer to this question is 'no' – there is no specific exemption because of a diagnosis of Parkinson's, although the Parkinson's Disease Society has been fighting for such an exemption for many years. However, many people with Parkinson's qualify for exemption from prescription charges on general grounds such as age, being in receipt of Income Support or being unable to collect their prescriptions themselves.

But this still leaves some younger people with Parkinson's, often on low incomes, struggling with heavy prescription costs. The only partial relief available in this situation is to pre-pay for your prescriptions by purchasing a 'season ticket', which can last for either four or 12 months and covers all the drugs you need during that period, not just the drugs for your Parkinson's. To apply, you need to fill in form FP95 available from most doctors' surgeries, from pharmacists, from Post Offices, or from the Family Health Service Authority. Before you go ahead, you need to do a careful calculation, based on the current price of ordinary prescriptions, the price of season tickets and your average number of prescriptions in a year, to see whether a season ticket will be helpful to you.

Other financial considerations

I was just about to buy a house when I was told I had Parkinson's. Will I be able to get a mortgage?

As with all decisions about mortgages, the answer will depend on your personal circumstances including your savings, income, likely security of employment (which may be affected by the diagnosis of Parkinson's) and on how much you want to borrow. Once you are sure in your own mind that you want to go ahead, you should shop around to see what various building societies and banks have on offer.

What attitude do life insurance companies take to a diagnosis of Parkinson's?

Life insurance companies normally ask people who wish to take out new policies to answer questions about their health or to undergo a medical examination. If these reveal a long-term condition like Parkinson's, the result can be either refusal or high premiums. However, there have recently been some widely publicised 'Over 50s' insurance schemes which guarantee acceptance without a medical or any questions. The benefits at death (after the first two years) are fixed amounts so if you live for many years, you could end up paying in more than the guaranteed benefit. You would however have several years of security, so such schemes may be worth considering if you feel that you are underinsured.

I am 55, married with a wife and two teenage children. I am considering retiring from work because of ill-health. What are the main economic factors which I should consider in making my decision?

You have not told us what your work is or which aspect of your Parkinson's is causing you to consider this course of action, so we can only give a general outline of the main considerations for anyone in this position. The important thing is not to rush into anything and to get as much information as possible about the choices open to you and about your likely sources of income.

First you need to consider whether you may, either now or in the future, consider a different kind of work. This might be full- or part-time and would be an especially important considera- tion for someone further away than you are from statutory retirement age. If this seems relevant, you should discuss the principle of other kinds of work and their likely effect on your health with your GP. If some alternative type of work is a likely option, then we would suggest you read the section on **Work** in Chapter 7.

Secondly you need to consider the practical route by which your retirement can be achieved. Once you and your GP are agreed that your health problems mean that you will be physically or mentally incapable of further work, you need to discover how the arrangements for your retirement can be made and how they will affect your future income.

If you have any doubts about your employer's attitude, it may be best to start with your union or professional body. If you are not a member of such an organisation, you could contact your local Citizens' Advice Bureau (see your local phone book for the address and telephone number). Although most employers are helpful, do remember that, irrespective of any health problem, you have the right not to be unfairly dismissed. If you have been continually employed by your present employer for two years or more, you have the right to pursue any dissatisfaction about the manner in which your employment ends through an industrial tribunal.

Assuming that your employer is one of the many who are

helpful, you should discuss the matter with him or her. In many instances, early retirement can be arranged with their full co-operation and support. Where occupational pension schemes are involved, they may, for example, assist employees to decide the most favourable route and timing for retirement. Details of any company pension scheme are usually available from your personnel department or directly from the pension company.

Thirdly you need to consider the full financial implications of giving up work. Your present and future financial commitments will be one part of the calculation, as will the question of whether your wife goes out to work or may do so in the future. If you have an occupational pension, you will still be eligible for the various non-means-tested benefits. Then, depending on your contributions record and degree of disability, you may be eligible for Incapacity Benefit (which has replaced both Invalidity Benefit and Sickness Benefit), Severe Disablement Allowance or Disability Living Allowance (see the section on *Benefits* earlier in this chapter for more information about these).

If you are not eligible for an occupational pension, then you may be eligible for some means-tested benefits such as Income Support, Housing Benefit and Council Tax Benefit. Eligibility for Income Support opens up access to other sorts of help such as free prescriptions, free dental treatment and free school meals for your children. Every type of benefit has its own qualifying conditions so it is very important to seek advice about the likely situation for your own individual circumstances. This can be obtained from the Benefits Agency, the Citizens' Advice Bureau (see your local phone book for address and phone numbers for both organisations), a welfare rights office (check with your local authority) or from the Welfare and Benefits Adviser at the Parkinson's Disease Society (see Appendix 1 for the address and phone number).

Can I get financial assistance from anywhere other than the Benefits Agency?

You may be able to get assistance for specific purposes such as help with the purchase of a particular item of equipment or a holiday from funds held by trade unions, professional organisations, Services' benevolent funds, local and national charitable trusts, churches and so on. The range of possible sources and of the conditions placed on recipients of grants varies enormously but usually you have to establish some personal connection. There is a book called the *Charities Digest* (your local library should have a reference copy) which lists many of these funds, and some Councils of Voluntary Service now have computer programs which can save you time by helping to identify the most likely sources for any particular set of circumstances. (If there is nothing listed under Council of Voluntary Service in your local phone book, then ask at your local Citizens' Advice Bureau about any local groupings of voluntary organisations which may be able to help in this way.) These organisations and your local library may also have a copy of a directory called *A Guide to Grants for Individuals in Need* (see Appendix 2 for details). It contains a comprehensive list of charities and organisations which can provide funds and the circumstances in which they might do so.

The Parkinson's Disease Society has a staff member (who can be contacted at the National Office) who specialises in helping people with Parkinson's to find sources of financial help.

As mentioned in the section on **Work** in Chapter 7, help with equipment which will help you obtain or retain employment is also available from the Department of Employment, as is help with the cost of journeys to work.

My husband is becoming very confused and is now unable to handle his financial affairs. Is there some way that I can be authorised to act for him?

This is quite a complex area of the law, and we would recommend that you discuss your situation with someone at the Citizens' Advice Bureau (see your local phone book for the address and phone number). They will be able to tell you if you need advice from a solicitor. Before you take any action, you may find it useful to read Age Concern's *Factsheet Number 22: Legal Arrangements for Managing Financial Affairs*. There is a version for England and Wales, and another - with the same number - for Scotland (where the law is different). You can obtain copies from the relevant Age Concern offices (the addresses and phone numbers are in Appendix 1). The fact sheets set out the various options which range from simple permissions to cash Social Security benefits to the legal documents required in cases of proven mental incapacity.

If your husband still has times when he is able to understand what he is doing, then you should discuss with him as soon as possible the idea of making an Enduring Power of Attorney. This is a legal document which allows him to appoint one or more persons to act for him. The document has to be drawn up on a special form and signed by both the donor (your husband) and the attorney (yourself and any others he appoints – the 'attorney' in a Power of Attorney does not mean a lawyer, although he could appoint a solicitor as his attorney if he wished to do so). It has to be completed while your husband is able to understand what he is signing. If he then becomes incapable of managing his own affairs, you apply to the Court of Protection (part of the Supreme Court) for registration of your Power of Attorney and you are then authorised to act for him without his consent. While you are organising your Power of Attorney you could also encourage your husband to make a will if he has not already made one.

If your husband is already too confused to understand what is involved in making an Enduring Power of Attorney, you will have to apply to the Court of Protection to be appointed as a Receiver (or, in Scotland, a Curator Bonum) for your husband's affairs. This is a more complex and costly procedure than making a Power of Attorney so it is certainly advisable to act sooner rather than later if at all possible.

12

Care outside the home

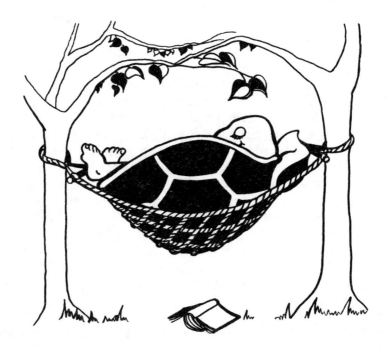

Introduction

As with most other sections of the population, the vast majority of people with Parkinson's spend most of their time at home. However sometimes, from choice or necessity, they spend some time outside the home and this chapter is about the variety of circumstances and locations in which this can occur. Except for holidays or respite care facilities which cater for couples, most of these situations involve the separation of the person with

Parkinson's from their carer and so can create anxieties for both parties. People differ greatly in their needs and choices and the range of provision can vary greatly from one area to another, so our answers can only indicate the likely solutions and suggest ways of following them up.

Respite care

What is respite care?

Respite care is any facility or resource which allows those who care for sick, frail, elderly or disabled relatives or friends to have a break from their caring tasks. Such breaks do not come as a right as holidays do with a paid job but they are equally, if not more, important and necessary.

There is a very useful publication called *Taking a Break* (see Appendix 2 for details of how to obtain a free copy) which discusses the various alternatives and deals sensitively and sympathetically with the fears and concerns which thoughts of respite care can sometimes arouse. It also has lots of examples of how very helpful and successful taking a break can be.

I don't want to go away but would like the occasional day or half-day to recharge my batteries and keep me sane. Do you know anywhere I can get this?

In the section on *Caring for the carers* in Chapter 5, we discussed how help could be brought into the home through schemes like Crossroads Care. Such schemes are, of course, an important way of having a break, although they tend to be for a few hours rather than a whole day.

You should contact your Social Services department to see what sort of respite services they offer. Some have Family Link schemes whereby another family will agree to take your relative into their home on a regular basis - for a few hours, a day, a weekend or even longer. All Social Services departments have some day centres offering company, meals, activities and supervision; they will also know about any similar facilities in your area provided by voluntary organisations such as the Red Cross and the Women's Royal Voluntary Service. Day centres cannot usually cope with severely disabled people, but there are other alternatives such as day hospitals (especially if some re-assessment or treatment is required) and day care in residential or nursing homes.

An approach via Social Services will be a useful first step, as they should assess the needs of your relative and yourself, take into account your wishes and preferences, and suggest what is available and what it will cost. Perhaps you should not exclude the possibility of a longer break which could be good for both of you. It will not hurt to know what is available.

I really want to continue looking after my wife but feel the need for regular breaks to keep me going. What is available?

Regular breaks can make an important contribution to people's ability to go on caring for their relatives. One major determinant of what is available is the type of care which your wife needs. If she does not require skilled nursing or special equipment, she may be able to have a regular break (how often depends on your needs and local resources) in a local authority or private residential home. If you think this is likely to be a suitable solution, approach your Social Services department with your request. They should assess your situation and tell you what is available to meet your needs. If your need is very urgent, your choice of places may be very restricted; with more time to plan, you would hope to have some choice. There will be a charge related to your ability to pay.

If your wife is severely disabled and needs nursing care, you may be able to arrange for her to go into hospital (usually in the care of a geriatrician) while you have a break. Depending on the level of need and the availability of local resources, the fre-quency of such admissions can vary from once a year up to every few weeks. You need to ask your GP if you want this kind of respite care. There is no charge for hospital care but, in some circumstances, benefits and allowances may be affected.

I don't know what to do. I am at my wits' end and feel in need of a break but my husband gets upset if I mention it and I am not sure that anyone else could look after him properly anyway.

Your distress and ambivalent feelings are shared by many people who have been caring for a relative for many years and are entirely understandable – as is your husband's anxiety about being cared for by someone else. It is a start to have put your feelings into words and now you need someone with whom you can explore them further. It will help if this person is someone who understands about Parkinson's and who also knows what options are open to you. You could talk to your doctor, to someone from Social Services, a community nurse or, if there is a local branch of the Parkinson's Disease Society nearby, one of their welfare visitors.

You are almost certainly correct in thinking that no-one will be able to look after your husband as well as you do but, by having a break, you will probably be able to carry on caring for him for longer, which is what you both want. You may also find that your husband is quite worried about you and that it will be easier for him to think through the problem if someone else is involved in the discussions. Try to find out as much as you can about any places which are suggested and visit them if at all possible. In this way, you can see for yourself what standard of service is being offered.

Is there anywhere I can go with my mother so that we both get a break but don't have to be separated?

Unfortunately not at present, although the Parkinson's Disease Society are trying to set up suitable facilities, in conjunction with various health trusts and similar care providers. The Society's newletter will carry full details when such accommodation becomes available.

If your mother is well enough to have a holiday rather than respite care, then we suggest you read the section on *Holidays* later in this chapter.

Going into hospital

My wife has to go into hospital shortly. Her speech is now very indistinct and she is used to having me on hand all day. I understand her needs and what she can and cannot do. Is there some way I can pass on this information without seeming to interfere?

Going into hospital creates anxiety for most people even if they are able to communicate easily, so you are very wise to think ahead about your wife's special needs. Copies of the simple information form shown in Figure 10 can be obtained from the Parkinson's Disease Society (address in Appendix 1). By completing one of these forms (or something similar), you can share your understanding of your wife's needs with the nursing staff. We are sure that they will find such information very useful. Many hospitals now have a named nurse or a small team of nurses allocated to each patient and it would obviously be a good idea to discuss the completed form with the named nurse or team leader when your wife is admitted.

If your wife uses a portable communication aid, make sure that she takes it with her to hospital. If she does not currently have a communication aid, it would be worth contacting the speech and language therapy department at the hospital to see if they can recommend one which would be suitable for her.

I have to go into hospital soon for an operation and need my Parkinson's medication at irregular hours. I would feel much less anxious if I knew that I could keep my tablets and take them when I need them. Will this be allowed or can they insist that I hand them over?

Your anxiety at the thought of not being able to have your tablets when you need them is shared by many people with Parkinson's who know only too well that sometimes even a few minutes can make a big difference. Hospital wards, especially non-neurological wards, are not generally geared up for people with very individual medication timetables and there have been many accounts of problems arising from this. However there is

INFORMATION FOR USE ON ADMISSION TO HOSPITAL

If you suffer from Parkinson's disease and are to be admitted to hospital for any reason, you may find it useful to complete this form giving details of your drug regime together with any other information about your personal needs which you consider would be helpful to the nursing staff responsible for your care

---

DETAILS OF PERSONAL CARE:

Name:_____   Date:_____

MEDICATION:
The following drugs (s) have been prescribed.
It is important that the following medicine (s) be taken at the times indicated.

Doses and times

Drug 1_____

Drug 2_____

Drug 3_____

Drug 4_____

Drug 5_____

(Doctor's Signature)_____Date:_____

ACTIVITY   ASSISTANCE REQUIRED/AIDS USED

Speech_____

Comprehension _____

Eating/Drinking_____

Walking_____

Washing/Bathing_____

Dressing _____

Bowels/Bladder_____

Other Information_____

(please continue on the back of this form, if necessary)

Figure 10: Information form for use on admission to hospital

a growing awareness of the serious difficulties which standard drug rounds (when the nurses give out medication at set times and not otherwise) cause for people with Parkinson's and some hospital wards are experimenting with self-medication (see Appendix 2 for details of Bernadette Porter's essay on this topic, which won the 'Mali Jenkins Medical Essay Prize' and is published by the Parkinson's Disease Society).

You should discuss your wish to retain control of your medication with the hospital consultant and the ward sister and see if you can come to a satisfactory arrangement. If not, you will almost certainly have to hand over your tablets. In this case, be sure to complete and hand over the information sheet shown in Figure 10 and discussed in our answer to the previous question.

My wife is due to go into hospital for a hysterectomy and I am worried because I have heard that the anaesthetic may upset her Parkinson's medication. Is this true and can anything be done to prevent it?

It is not so much that the anaesthetic 'upsets' the Parkinson's medication as that operations under anaesthetic require that anything taken by mouth (food or drink or medicine) has to be withdrawn shortly before the operation. This causes very understandable anxiety to people like your wife who depend on their medication for reasonable mobility and comfort.

Do talk to the medical and nursing staff on her ward so that they understand how important your wife's Parkinson's medication is, and ask them to withdraw it for the shortest possible time. It may also be worth remembering that injections of apomorphine can be used to 'rescue' people with Parkinson's from severe episodes of immobility at times when taking medication by mouth is not possible. If there is a local Parkinson's Nurse Specialist, you could perhaps ask her to liaise with the staff on the ward.

My husband (aged 79 and suffering from Parkinson's) was poorly treated and neglected whilst in hospital recently. How can I complain?

We are very sorry to learn of your husband's unhappy experience and would certainly encourage you to make a complaint.

All hospitals (and Social Services departments) now have to have complaints procedures and to make them known to the public. Many have special leaflets which set out what action you should take and whom you can contact, either to make the complaint yourself or to get help and support in making it.

In general, our advice would be that if you are concerned about any aspect of health service provision then you should discuss your concern, as soon as possible, with the person who gave (or failed to give) the service in question. Sometimes misunderstandings or disagreements can be sorted out in this direct face-to-face way. If you are nervous or uncertain, take a friend or relative with you.

If this action leaves you dissatisfied, you can get help from your local Community Health Council (see your local phone book for the address and telephone number). The Community Health Council is an independent voice on health issues in the local community and it also helps individuals, like you, who want to make a complaint. They understand how the procedures work and will help you to think through your options, prepare your evidence and, if you wish, arrange for someone to accompany you at meetings with hospital managers.

Do not be afraid to make your complaint. Even though your husband's unhappy experience cannot be changed now, you can alert the hospital to the problem and so help to improve standards for other users. There are three golden rules for anyone wanting to make a complaint: complain as soon as possible after the incident, be courteous, and provide accurate details of the incident such as date, time, place and people involved.

My father is in hospital and I am worried that they will discharge him without sufficient help. He lives near me but is unrealistic about what he can do for himself. I supervise and do some meals but can only do a certain amount because I also have to care for my disabled husband. What should I do?

Mention your concerns to the ward sister immediately and ask to see a social worker. Since April 1993, every hospital and its local Social Services department has had to have an approved hospital discharge agreement. This is meant to ensure that people like your father are not sent back home without adequate services. If he has complex needs, he should receive a full community care assessment (see Chapter 4 for more information about these) which should also include an assessment of your needs as his carer. Stick to your guns and insist that he is given this assessment, and remember that you also have the right to comment on its findings. If the result of the assessment is a recommendation for residential or nursing home care, there is further relevant information in the next section.

Long-term care

How do I find the right residential or nursing home accommodation for my needs?

First you need to be sure what your needs are and whether you want to opt for permanent care outside your own home. Knowing the type of care you require will help you to decide whether you could remain at home if you wished to do so or, if you could not, whether you need residential home or nursing home care. Another important element in the equation is your age and whether or not you have a spouse who also has some care needs.

Do try to talk the whole question over from every possible angle with someone you trust – deciding on permanent care is a very important decision and not one to be taken lightly.

If you have family and friends near your present home, you will probably want to stay in the same area. Unless you are able to pay the full cost of your care for several years, you will need your local Social Services to agree that you are in need of long-term care. You should therefore contact the department and ask for an assessment. They will provide a written report with which you can agree or disagree.

Whether you need financial assistance or not, you need to find out what is available. Your local Social Services department and Health Authority will have lists of all registered homes in the area and some information about size and facilities. However there is no substitute for visiting the homes and seeing things for yourself. Do ask questions (see the next answer for some suggestions) – of the staff, of the residents and of their relatives. Local professional workers and volunteers may also have useful comments and experiences to add to your own researches.

If, alternatively, you want to move to another part of the country, perhaps to be near a relative, you need to make the same sort of enquiries in that area. If you are likely to need financial assistance, you will still have to involve the Social Services department for the place where you live now.

In circumstances where the type or quality of care is more important than its location – perhaps because you are relatively young or have particular problems in controlling your Parkinson's symptoms – there are a few other options. One might be a home like those owned and run by the Leonard Cheshire Foundation which tend to have younger residents; another might be the new residential home for people with Parkinson's in Walsall (see Appendix 1 for relevant addresses). Nearly all such homes have waiting lists and you will need to take this into account when making your plans.

What sort of questions should I have in mind when viewing a residential or nursing home?

Just as in thinking about moving to a new house, the potential list of questions is very long indeed! We have tried to highlight a few key areas.

The first crucially important questions are about the type and quality of medical, nursing and specialist care available. This will relate mainly to your present needs but it will be worth enquiring what will happen if you need additional care in the future. You may want to know whether you can keep your own doctor (if he or she is willing to visit) and whether dentists, opticians and therapists make regular visits to the home.

Secondly you need to consider the nature and quality of the

accomodation. You could ask questions about its overall size, whether there is a choice of single or shared rooms, the availability of sitting and recreation rooms, the standard and variety of washing and bathroom facilities, ease of access including ramps and lifts, and whether there are special arrangements or rules about smoking or pets.

Your third area of interest is the general atmosphere. Are the staff welcoming but also open to questions? Do the other residents look well cared for, comfortable and interested in what is going on? Is there sufficient privacy? Are there facilities for visitors to stay overnight?

Location is another important topic. If you wish to remain in the area which you know well in order to keep in touch with family, friends, particular facilities like church, shops or meeting places, then this will be a crucial consideration for you. Alternatively you may wish to move to another district or town to be close to relatives or friends or you may wish to live in a particular home where you already have friends or contacts. On a more general level, you may prefer a quiet, rural location or a busy, urban one.

Some Health Authorities and Social Services departments now provide leaflets containing general advice and questions such as the ones we have mentioned. It would be worth finding out if something like this is available where you live, as you could then take it along with you when visiting any potential homes. Two other useful checklists of relevant questions are Counsel and Care's *Factsheet Number 5: What to look for in a Private or Voluntary Registered Home* and *Which?* magazine's article *Choosing a Care Home* (see Appendix 2 for further details of both these publications).

What if the place I like charges more than I can afford from my own income?

If your income and savings are greater than the maximum allowed under current government regulations (you can check what this is by contacting your local Social Services department or Benefits Agency) then you would not be eligible for help from Social Services. In these circumstances you would have to see if what you can afford in fees could be topped up from elsewhere – for example by a relative, or by a grant from a charity or benevolent fund on which you have some call. If, on the other hand, your income and capital are below the cut-off level, and you have been assessed as needing the type of care provided by this particular home, and the costs do not exceed those normally allowed by Social Services for such care, then any shortfall will be met by the Social Services department.

The Social Services department, the Citizens' Advice Bureau and the Parkinson's Disease Society (address in Appendix 1) will be able to offer more specific advice related to your individual circumstances.

My father was taken into hospital after a fall when he broke his hip. He is now very confused and I am told that he must go into a private nursing home. Can they do this?

There is no simple answer to this question, as you have touched on one of the least clear areas of health policy. The main unresolved issues concern the distinction between 'treatment' and 'care' and there are no easy solutions which would be both practical, affordable and equitable between individuals.

Until recently our view was that you could not legally be forced to move your father to a private nursing home but, at the time of writing, new guidelines for hospitals and Social Services departments are being prepared and the position seems likely to change. If your hospital authority has no continuous care beds (see the *Glossary* for a definition of these), it is very likely that you will have difficulty in insisting that your father remains on an acute ward. The cause of your father's confusion, whether or not it can be treated, and the outlook for his physical health are all important components in the picture and could affect the outcome.

If your father has not already had a community care assessment (see Chapter 4 for more details), you should request one (through the ward staff or Social Services) immediately. The nature of your father's care needs will then become clearer and you can be involved in discussions about alternative solutions.

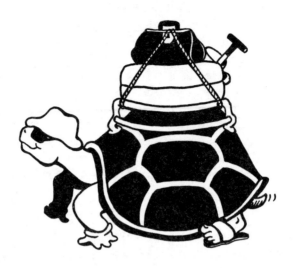

Holidays

My husband and I have not had a holiday for years because of my Parkinson's - really I have lost confidence. Could you suggest anything which would be suitable?

It is easy to lose confidence when you have not been away for a long time but take your courage in both hands because there are a whole range of possibilities. First you need to decide between yourselves what sort of holiday you would like and how far you want to travel. Think about how much care and attention you need and whether you want to have access to particular activities or pastimes.

When you have sorted out your own ideas, you need to discuss your options with someone who knows what is available. If you happen to have a local branch of the Parkinson's Disease Society, they may be able to help. Otherwise you could contact the Holidays Organiser at the Parkinson's Disease Society's National Office (see Appendix 1 for the address and phone number, or for similar details of the other national organisations mentioned in this answer). There are also two national organisations which provide information and advice about holidays for people with special needs. They are the Holiday Care Service which can suggest particular places and advise about transport, insurance and people to contact for help in meeting the cost of a holiday; and RADAR (Royal Association for Disability and Rehabilitation) which produces very informative guides on holidays in the British Isles and abroad.

If you have a particular resort in mind, it would be worth contacting their information office, as many holiday resorts produce special information about accommodation and facilities for people with disabilities. Your local Social Services department may also have some general information. In some towns there are travel agents or coach operators who offer special holidays for people with mobility problems, so do ask around to find out if there is something like this in your locality.

If you would feel happier going with people who have specialised knowledge of Parkinson's, the Parkinson's Disease Society runs special holidays for couples each year at various locations around the country. There is also usually one holiday abroad. Some local branches of the Society also organise weekend or longer holidays.

One of the organisations used by the Parkinson's Disease Society for its special holidays is the Winged Fellowship Trust – a charity committed to providing real holidays for people with disabilities. It has purpose-built or specially adapted holiday homes which can cater for people with severe mobility problems and it recruits young volunteers who help to look after the holidaymakers and so ensure that they have a proper holiday.

If you are going abroad, either on an organised holiday or independently, remember to arrange adequate insurance cover (and to tell the insurance company about your Parkinson's). Medical attention is free in all European Union countries although you should obtain form number E111 (from the Post Office) before you go.

I need to get away for a break but would feel happier if my father, who has Parkinson's, could have a holiday rather than just go into a hospital or a home. What can you suggest?

Most of the organisations mentioned in the answer to the

previous question cater for people on their own. The Winged Fellowship was founded to provide just the sort of thing you are looking for – a break for you and a real holiday for your father – and the Holiday Care Association has a service called Holiday Helpers which links people needing assistance with carefully selected volunteers. Some of the Parkinson's Disease Society's holidays are suitable for unaccompanied people with Parkinson's.

I would love a holiday but don't think that I could afford anywhere with the special facilities which I need. Are there any sources of financial help?

Yes there are, although your eligibility for help will depend on your personal circumstances. The Holiday Care Service (address in Appendix 1) can put enquirers in touch with possible sources of financial help. The Parkinson's Disease Society tries to ensure that no-one goes without a holiday because of a shortage of funds and they have a member of staff who is expert in identifying sources of help. Some towns have charitable funds for use by local residents (ask at your local authority offices or local library), and there are a large number of benevolent funds listed in two books which we have already mentioned in Chapter 11 – the *Charities Digest* and *A Guide to Grants for Individuals in Need* (your local library or Citizen's Advice Bureau should have reference copies).

13
Research and clinical trials

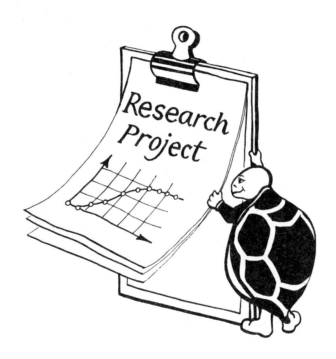

Introduction

Research – the careful and systematic search for answers – is very important for conditions such as Parkinson's for which there is currently no cure. Research is also important when (again as in Parkinson's) there are various treatments available, none of which is perfect.

In this chapter we consider three different aspects of research: medical research; the clinical trials which are a common feature of such research; and other research projects in related fields which can throw light on the management of Parkinson's, the delivery of services, and the overall quality of life of people with Parkinson's. Our aim is to give an overview of the state of research at the time this book was written. We do not claim that our answers are comprehensive, as new discoveries are taking place all the time and it is impossible to be completely up to date. The Parkinson's Disease Society has a special interest group for people who wish to keep up with medical research findings. The group is called Spring, and there is more information about it in Chapter 14.

Medical research

What progress is being made in identifying the cause of Parkinson's?

Before answering this question, it is worth us spending a little time recapping on the nature of Parkinson's. It is a degenerative disorder which becomes increasingly common with advancing age. The degeneration of nerve cells (this is defined in the *Glossary*) found in Parkinson's only occurs in one small part of the brain. This pattern of selective loss of cells is also found in other degenerative conditions, for example in Alzheimer's disease, motor neurone disease and the Parkinson's Plus syndromes. This similarity means that research findings in any one of these conditions may throw light on the causes of the other conditions as well.

One strand of research in Parkinson's is concerned with the scars or marks (called Lewy bodies) which are left when nerve cells die. Understanding the proteins which make up these microscopic structures may turn out to be very important.

In the last few years more clues to the causes of Parkinson's have been discovered than ever before, thanks - perhaps surprisingly - to some American drug addicts! This modern era of research dates from about 10 years ago when a group of young drug addicts in America developed an illness that looked just like Parkinson's. They had taken a drug of abuse containing MPTP. The chemical involved in this drug is a relatively simple one, and it came as a great surprise to researchers to find that such a drug could cause the death of those specific nerve cells that are affected in Parkinson's whilst leaving the rest of the brain and body alone.

Researchers then discovered that MPTP can cause Parkinson's in monkeys so, for the first time, they had an animal model to help test their theories. (We recognise that some people have strongly held views both for and against the use of animals in medical research, but we do not think that a book of this type is the right place to explore such controversies.) MPTP was found to damage particular parts of the cell called the mitochondria – the energy pack of the cell. When the mitochondria fail, a number of other biochemical processess also fail and lead to the death of the nerve cell. It was also thought that chemicals like MPTP might produce other compounds called 'oxygen free radicals' which are known to have the ability to cause cell damage. Studies done on postmortem samples of brain from people with Parkinson's have provided evidence that both mitochondrial damage and activation of free radicals do indeed occur. These are important clues which may lead researchers closer to the cause of Parkinson's.

One possibility is that there are other chemicals, perhaps in the environment or in food, which are rather like MPTP. Some people may have a genetically determined weakness in their defence system against chemicals which means that, unlike unaffected people, they are unable to break them down in their bodies into other harmless substances. The compounds could then cause damage to the substantia nigra (there is a diagram in Chapter 1 showing the position of the substantia nigra).

The availability of an animal model may also help researchers to identify ways in which the damage caused can be halted or even reversed. It has already helped with the development of new dopamine agonists (there is more information about these drugs in Chapter 3) and with the evaluation of foetal cell implants and other surgical procedures.

What areas of current Parkinson's research seem most encouraging?

Researchers are currently concentrating on four major areas: identifying people at risk; preventing further progression after diagnosis; repairing the damaged brain; and developing new drugs and operations.

Much current research is aimed at trying to find out whether or not we can identify people with Parkinson's before they ever get their first symptom, perhaps by using some form of biochemical test or some sort of scanning device. PET (positron emission tomography) scanning can show the loss of the dopamine cells and pathways in Parkinson's, but these machines are very expensive and there are currently only two in the whole of Britain. Knowledge of how cell damage occurs might help us to prevent symptoms emerging in those people shown to be vulnerable, either by improving their defences or by helping them avoid whatever was likely to trigger the appearance of symptoms.

Such understanding of the mechanisms of nerve cell damage may also allow us to prevent further deterioration in people who already have early symptoms. After all, most people are only mildly affected when they are first diagnosed, so if we could just hold it at that point, much would be achieved.

Methods of repairing brains which are already seriously damaged by Parkinson's are another avenue for research. The most publicised procedure is that using foetal brain cells (discussed in the next few questions) but there are other, more distant possibilities. These include the use of other types of cells which have been genetically engineered to contain dopamine, or the identification of substances known as growth factors (see the *Glossary* for a definition) which could help the brain to repair itself.

The development of new drugs is a major research area. Researchers are looking for new ways of giving L-dopa supplements and attempting to develop new dopamine agonists which are as powerful as L-dopa replacement therapy (there is more information about currently available dopamine agonists in

Chapter 3). If such dopamine agonists could be developed, it might be possible to eliminate or prevent the fluctuations in response to drugs which we now sometimes see after people have been on treatment for several years. Operations such as pallidotomy (discussed in the section on *Surgical treatments* in Chapter 3) are also a very active area of research.

I watched a programme on TV about foetal implants. Can you explain how significant these have been and whether they hold out a real hope for people like me (I have had Parkinson's for 15 years)?

Foetal implants have certainly hit the headlines. They are experimental procedures that may or may not have a good future. Only a few people across the whole world appear to have shown any useful degree of improvement after such an implant.

Different ways of doing the operation (including variations in the type of cells implanted) are under very active investigation. Researchers are keen to carry on with these investigations because the response in animals has been good. Animals, however, do not have Parkinson's itself but only a simulated form of the condition. Translating the good animal response to foetal implants into good results in human beings who actually have the disease may take several more years of research.

Will these developments hold out any hope for people like you? In reply we can only say that any good new treatment for Parkinson's (including implants that really work) will probably be effective in anyone whose Parkinson's is uncomplicated by other problems, no matter how many years have passed since diagnosis.

How do I go about being considered for a foetal implant operation?

The way your question is worded suggests that you are thinking of this operation as a treatment for your symptoms. At the moment, as explained in the answer to the previous question, such operations are experimental and because of this are, quite rightly, not available as treatment either on the NHS or in the private sector. The people who have had the operations are those who have fulfilled certain requirements specified by the researchers and who have been willing to act as experimental subjects. If you are seriously interested in accepting such a role with all its associated risks, you should talk to your own neurologist about where teams working in this area of research are based (at present there are none in this country). You should also discuss the pros and cons of such a course of action.

I have moral objections to abortion so would feel unable to accept surgery using foetal tissue. What are the chances of ethically acceptable implant material becoming available?

With current advances in genetic engineering it is quite possible that in the foreseeable future cells for use as implant material will be derived from sources other than aborted foetuses. They might, for example, come from normal skin and be 'engineered' to produce dopamine or growth factors (see the *Glossary* for definitions). Cells that produce growth factors may turn out to be just as important as dopamine producing cells in our search to find ways of repairing damaged brains.

I have heard that Parkinson's drugs could be given by patches on the skin which deliver several doses before having to be replaced. Such a method could be a boon for rather forgetful older people. How soon might this option become a reality?

Skin patches have, as you probably know, proved useful in the treatment of some other conditions such as angina (which affects the heart). Delivery of Parkinson's drugs using skin patches is already available for some anticholinergic drugs, and has certainly been considered for other drugs as such a system might address the serious problems created by the levels of dopamine in the blood going up and down too quickly. So far most of these attempts are still at the experimental stage.

Although we cannot offer a definite time scale, we think that patches for Parkinson's drugs may become available within the next few years. They may deliver one of the currently used drugs or - and perhaps more likely - a new drug. As you suggest, patches could be very helpful for people who are rather forgetful but, more importantly, they may help to reduce the fluctuations in response to medication which people find so distressing.

Clinical trials

How can I find out what drug trials are taking place and whether I am eligible to participate?

We suggest you find out which doctors in your area are particularly interested in Parkinson's. These doctors (who may be either neurologists or specialists in the care of the elderly) are the ones who are most likely to be involved in carrying out drug trials from time to time. As all drug trials require their volunteers to return to hospital for quite frequent assessments, it is not sensible to get involved in drug trials outside your own area.

Eligibility to take part will vary from one trial to another depending on the type of drug and the questions which the researchers are trying to answer. For example, some drug trials need volunteers who have not yet started on drug treatment for their Parkinson's. Other trials may be trying out new dopamine agonists (there is more information about dopamine agonists in Chapter 3), and for these the researchers usually need people who have been on L-dopa for a number of years and who are beginning to develop fluctuating responses to their present treatment.

As well as these 'trial-specific eligibility criteria', there are some more general exclusion criteria which rule out certain groups of people for their own safety. You will usually find that such excluded groups include women who are likely to become pregnant, people with other serious conditions such as heart disease or dementia, and people who are extremely old.

While we applaud your wish to help with research, we would urge you to remember that taking part in a drug trial is not something which should be undertaken without careful consideration – the next two questions raise some of the points which you should consider before agreeing to take part.

I am very disabled and very frustrated, so I do not see why I should not be allowed to try some of the more experimental drugs. However, it seems that you always have to agree that you may get the placebo. That is no good to me – I have no time to wait.

Although in general there are many drug trials which use placebos, they are in fact rather rare in trials for Parkinson's drugs. Most recent Parkinson's drug trials have compared the new drug being tested with the best of the currently available treatments (such as Sinemet, Madopar or a dopamine agonist). So in these trials everyone is receiving an active treatment.

However, to complete the picture, we will explain why placebos are used in some instances. It is important to realise that experimental drugs are unproven. Nobody knows if they are going to work or, if they do work, in whom – or if they will have any unwanted side effects. If it was already known that the drug was effective and safe, it would not be necessary to carry out such trials. As it is difficult for either the volunteer (who badly wants an improved drug) or the investigator (who badly wants this new drug to be successful) to be totally objective, it is often necessary to compare the new drug with a placebo (a tablet which looks the same, is harmless, but has no active ingredients). The experimental drug and the placebo have to be allocated 'blind', which means they are given out in a way which ensures that neither the volunteer (as you note in your question) nor the investigator knows who has had which tablet.

When responses to the drug and the placebo are compared at the end of the trial, it is then possible to judge whether the experimental drug has had any real effect. If it is shown to be effective and to have no significant side effects, then it may well become a drug that is used for treatment. We would therefore like to assure you that if you are asked to take part in a drug trial with a placebo, it is because the researchers truly do not know whether the new drug will help you, will make no difference to you, or will even make you worse.

My husband's neurologist is very involved in research and

often asks for volunteers. What questions should we ask to ensure that we make the right decisions for ourselves?

People with Parkinson's may be asked to volunteer for several types of research. At the simplest level, there may be requests for a one-off test such as a blood or urine sample. These involve no risk or major discomfort or inconvenience so, if you are satisfied with the reason given for the request, you should be able to decide quite quickly between yourselves whether or not to take part.

The most likely request for volunteers is for participation in a drug trial. More is involved here and you are very sensible to think about the information you need to help you decide about taking part. First of all you need a proper explanation of the reason for the drug trial, and you should receive this both in a face-to-face discussion with your doctor or the researcher and also in writing. You should not be asked to make an immediate decision at the end of the discussion, but if you are, you should say that you want more time to consider.

During this discussion you can also raise any questions you have, both about the drug being tested and about practical matters to do with the trial. We list some of the more obvious questions here, but you will probably want to add others of your own.

- Has the drug been given to people with Parkinson's before? If it has, to how many and with what results? (If the results were encouraging, you are more likely to want to take part in a further test.)
- What, if any, side effects can you expect? (Any side effects will probably only be minor, as both the drug company and your local ethics committee will have reassured themselves that no serious side effects are likely. Your local ethics committee is made up of medical professionals and lay people from your area, and they are responsible for approving all the medical research that takes place within your Health Authority.)
- Will taking part in the trial cause you any inconvenience?
- How often will you have to return to hospital for tests?
- Will you receive travel expenses?

- How long will the tests and examinations take each time and what will be involved?
- Will the tests be physical examinations, blood tests, psychological tests or something else entirely?

Armed with this information and the written description of the trial, you should then consider your options for a day or two and, if possible, discuss the issues with someone who is approachable and reasonably knowledgeable. This could be your GP or a research nurse, nurse practitioner or Parkinson's Nurse Specialist at the hospital. You can then go back to your doctor or the researcher with any further questions and your decision. Deciding to take part does not commit you to staying in the trial until it is completed – you have the right to withdraw at any time and for any reason (or even for no reason at all).

Many people get a great deal of satisfaction from taking part in research, and doctors and researchers certainly appreciate the co-operation of people with Parkinson's. However, it is important that people take a thoughtful approach, as you are doing, and that they do not feel pressurised in any way to join in a trial or to stay in it if they wish to withdraw.

What protection do volunteers have against injury or illness resulting from participation in clinical trials?

It is of course true that there is a small but significant element of risk in any experimental procedure. However, if no risks were ever taken, we would not be able to make progress in research. The important thing is that the risks should be kept to a minimum (through careful application of agreed procedures by the drug companies, the ethics committees and the researchers) and that, as discussed in the previous question, potential volunteers should have full information about the possible risks. Although there have recently been some examples of trials of surgical experiments (where the risks are somewhat higher), most Parkinson's clinical trials will be drug trials. All participants are closely monitored and the results communicated to other interested parties so, if unexpected and undesirable side effects appear, rapid action can be taken.

Before being included in a clinical trial, you will have to sign a consent form stating that you understand what is involved and agree to take part. If there is anything on the consent form which you do not understand, ask. Do not sign until you understand.

You do not mention compensation for distress or suffering arising from unexpected side effects, but to complete the picture, we should mention that there is an agreement covering such rare events between the drug companies and the Health Authorities.

I have heard about requests for donations to the Brain Bank. What is it and what does a donation involve?

The Parkinson's Disease Society's Brain Tissue Bank (to give it its full name) was founded in 1984 to provide a new and important resource for research into Parkinson's. Ordinary 'high street' banks are places where people deposit their money and where skilled bankers use the accumulated wealth to create yet more wealth. The same sort of principles operate in a tissue bank, except that in this case only a promise is required during someone's life. Then at death, when the body may seem useless, it suddenly acquires new value as part of the Brain Tissue Bank's deposits. From these deposits new wealth will emerge in the form of greater understanding of Parkinson's and, we hope, discovery of its cause.

Researchers have already made major contributions to our understanding of Parkinson's by using samples of brain and other tissues provided by the Bank. They include researchers from many other parts of the world as well as those working at the Bank and at other centres in Britain.

For the Brain Tissue Bank to succeed, four different groups of people need to be involved.

1. People (both those with Parkinson's and others who do not have Parkinson's) who are willing to donate their brains or brains plus other organs, and relatives who are willing to carry out their wishes.
2. Specialists in Parkinson's who are willing to give their time to

seeing Parkinson's donors and to keeping careful records of their symptoms and treatment over the years between donation and death.

3. Research scientists who will study the brains and other tissues alongside the detailed medical information collected during life.

4. GPs who will discuss the project with interested people and be the links between donors and their relatives, specialists and Brain Tissue Bank staff.

The importance of good links between the groups becomes especially clear when death occurs because, to be really useful, the relevant tissues have to be removed quickly – within about six hours.

All these matters are dealt with in much more detail in the pamphlets produced by the Brain Tissue Bank which can be obtained from the address given in Appendix 1.

Other areas of research

I have found that the physical therapies (I mean physiotherapy, occupational therapy and speech and language therapy) make an important contribution to my well-being. Is any research taking place in these areas?

There has been growing interest in research into these therapies in recent years, partly because – helpful as the drugs are – many people with Parkinson's still have some problems even when they are on the best possible drug treatment. A big problem in planning research into these therapies is that double-blind trials (see the **Glossary** for a definition of these) are not possible, as you cannot pretend to give someone physiotherapy or speech exercises! It is also difficult to gather together large groups of people whose medication will remain unchanged during the time it takes to complete the research.

In spite of these problems some interesting studies have been done to identify particular methods of treatment for problems such as small steps, hurrying gait, freezing in doorways, speech problems and facial immobility.

Another strand of research has looked at the availability of these services, and has found evidence both of lack of referrals to therapists and of shortage of resources. These studies, and the pressure from people with Parkinson's and their relatives, have almost certainly helped to increase awareness of the contribution made by these therapies. There are now more therapists around the country with a special interest in Parkinson's, a development which has been encouraged by working parties in physiotherapy and speech therapy set up and funded by the Parkinson's Disease Society.

Other studies have looked at the best ways of delivering these services (for example, at home rather than in hospitals), and at ways of involving carers and so improving the likelihood that exercises will be continued and good habits maintained when the visits to the therapist come to an end.

Have there been any studies about the overall management of Parkinson's?

Yes, there have been a good many. This type of research really began in the late 1970s, when the Parkinson's Disease Society conducted a study of the people with Parkinson's who were then in touch with the Society. This study helped to identify important areas of unmet need – for information, therapy, welfare support, transport and company. Since then there have been several different projects which have focused on particular aspects of need.

An early project looked at how the work of the Society's branches could be improved and made more effective. From this study came the proposal that there should be professionally qualified regional support workers plus paid part-time welfare visitors. A follow-up study evaluated the work of the proposed regional staff in three different areas of the country.

Another project attempted to set up a model of good practice which would provide continuity of care, information and multi-disciplinary support, including careful consideration of how people are told about their diagnosis. It showed that such team support was acceptable to an unselected group of newly diagnosed people, that it responded to real needs in a flexible way and created a satisfying and viable way for staff to work together. This project, like a later one which concentrated on providing support and counselling around the time of diagnosis, catered for both people with Parkinson's and those with other long-term neurological conditions. A study which focused on communication between doctors and patients illustrated their differing attitudes to the diagnosis of Parkinson's and provided clues about how communication might be made more effective. Other studies have looked at the needs of people with Parkinson's living in the community, particularly those most seriously disabled, and at ways in which their needs could be met.

All these studies underline the need to listen to people with Parkinson's and to respond in ways appropriate to their individual needs.

Has there been any research addressed to the needs of people who care for those with Parkinson's?

All the studies mentioned in the answer to the previous question included attention to the needs of carers, but one particular research study has investigated the causes of stress in carers. This found that the main cause of stress was the occurrence of depression in the person with Parkinson's, and this finding has directed attention to the need for early diagnosis and treatment of depressive episodes. Other studies, started recently, are going to look at the ways in which psychological changes in people with Parkinson's affect their carers, and at the communication difficulties of people who have both Parkinson's and dementia and how their carers can be helped.

Have there been any research projects on aspects relevant to younger people with Parkinson's?

Yes. There was a study of the important topic of self-medication in hospital (an entry for the 'Mali Jenkins Medical Essay Prize' - details of the study are in Appendix 2) and a project which helped to set up a pilot driving test centre for people with disabilities (this centre has now become a permanent part of the national network of driving test centres). Preparations are in hand for a study which will explore the gynaecological problems encountered by women who have Parkinson's.

Another study of special interest to younger people was carried out for the Parkinson's Disease Society by the National Children's Bureau. It focused on the perceptions and experiences of the children of people with Parkinson's, and has led the Society to plan some publications about Parkinson's for children and teenagers.

The Parkinson's Disease Society

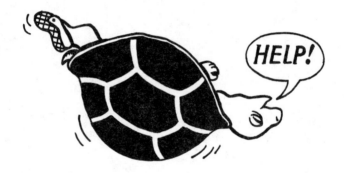

Introduction

We have frequently referred in this book to the Parkinson's Disease Society of the United Kingdom (PDS for short) - the UK voluntary organisation which is dedicated to helping people with Parkinson's. In this chapter we draw a fuller and more cohesive picture of the Society and the ways in which it helps and supports people with Parkinson's and those who care for them. It is a straightforward description of what is available and is not written as questions and answers.

Further information about the Parkinson's Disease Society, its branches and special interest groups can be obtained by filling in the form at the back of this book or simply by writing direct to the Society at the address in Appendix 1.

Aims and organisation

The Society was founded in 1969 by a very determined and charismatic lady called Miss Mali Jenkins. She had just retired when one of her sisters was diagnosed with Parkinson's and, finding that there was no society to offer information and advice or to support research, she set about filling the gap. The Society has three aims:

- to help patients and their relatives with the problems arising from Parkinson's;
- to collect and disseminate information on Parkinson's;
- to encourage and provide funds for research into Parkinson's.

The Society has thousands of members throughout the country and continues to welcome new members, but it exists to help and encourage all people with Parkinson's regardless of whether or not they are members. It has a National Office in London (address in Appendix 1) staffed by specialists in welfare, education and information, publicity and fundraising, research and general administration. There are field staff around the country who promote the Society and the needs of people with Parkinson's in their areas and who help to found and support branches of the Society.

Branches

The branches, of which there are over 200, are local self-help groups which offer opportunities for mutual support, emo-tional and practical help, social and educational activities and fundraising. They have good links with other organisations in their particular areas which can provide further help and advice on a whole variety of topics.

Although all branches arrange regular opportunities for members to meet each other both to exchange information and for recreation, it is important to understand that such meetings are only a part of branch activities, and that there is no obligation for you to attend them. Most branches try to respond to enquirers in whatever way is best suited to their individual needs and wishes, so it is perfectly possible to ask for written information, to exchange ideas or to ask questions over the phone, or to have a visit from a branch volunteer or welfare visitor.

An increasing number of branches are reaching out to people with Parkinson's by appointing welfare visitors, or by introducing innovative schemes such as day centres, drop-in centres or information courses for newly-diagnosed people. Other branches organise therapy sessions, or provide financial support or transport for courses organised by local health professionals. Some branches have their own minibus to help with transport needs, while others make use of community transport or assistance offered by other voluntary organisations. Improved access to respite care through contact or contracts with organisations such as Crossroads Care is a feature of some branches, while others organise branch holidays and mini-breaks. As you can see, the range of activities and support available is considerable!

As branches are mutual help organisations, many people join in the hope of serving others as well as helping themselves, and there is no shortage of things for them to do. As well as taking part in branch activities, either as committee members or in less public roles, branch members represent their branches at regional and national meetings of the Society and make invaluable contributions to the Society's education role. They can be found talking to local Women's Institutes and similar organisations, to schools, to health and social work professionals, and to many other groups who wish to know more about the complex and variable condition known as Parkinson's. Branch members may also take an active part with members of other voluntary groups in making the voice of the user and consumer of health and social services heard in discussions and decisions on such topics.

Welfare

The first aim of the Society – helping patients and their relatives with problems arising from Parkinson's – is mainly the responsibility of the Welfare Department, the field staff and the branches.

Counselling and the telephone Helpline

The Society has a counsellor who is able to provide a confidential service to people with problems and who also trains and supports the volunteers who staff the telephone Helpline.

This Helpline is available to anyone throughout the country and operates from 10.00 am to 4.00 pm on weekdays. It offers a totally confidential listening ear and can lead to further contact with workers in the Society or elsewhere who can offer relevant advice or help.

Benefits

The Welfare and Benefits Adviser helps to sort out complex benefits enquiries, advises those wishing to appeal against benefit or driving decisions and makes representations to statutory bodies about the general welfare needs of people with Parkinson's, for example community care, prescription charges and so on.

General help and advice

Information, advice and practical help concerning health and welfare services, transport, holidays, respite and long-term care are all available from the Welfare team and from workers in the branches. The Society organises some holidays itself each year but also has links with other organisations which provide holidays for people with mobility and other problems. The same is true for many other aspects of care – the Society can be a very good channel to other sources of help and advice in the voluntary, statutory and private sectors. The addresses and telephone numbers of many of these other organisations will be found in Appendix 1.

Education and information

The Society's second aim, the dissemination of information, is mainly the responsibility of the Education and Information Department.

The Education Officer plans and organises seminars and courses for professionals who care for people with Parkinson's, for branches, for staff and for members of the Society. The Information Officers reply to enquiries from members, professionals and the public and are building up the Society's library which, as well as a range of relevant books, contains Parkinson's newsletters from around the world.

Staff in the Education and Information Department produce a wide range of literature and videos to increase understanding of Parkinson's and its impact on people with Parkinson's and their carers. Many of the titles published by the Society are listed in Appendix 2, but you can get a complete list by writing direct to the Society at the address given in Appendix 1.

The Education and Information Department also takes an active part in the Society's efforts to raise public awareness of Parkinson's.

Research

Supporting research into Parkinson's, which is the Society's third aim, continues to have a high profile. The Society receives many applications for research grants, and the Medical and

Welfare Advisory Panels study these and make recommendations. Medical research has focused on understanding the
processes occuring in the brain, on searching for the cause of
Parkinson's, and on developing new and more effective treatments. Welfare research has included exploring better ways of
providing care for people with Parkinson's. Many of the research
projects mentioned in Chapter 13 have been supported by the
Parkinson's Disease Society. The Society also funds its own
Brain Tissue Bank (there is more information about this in
Chapter 13).

Fundraising

Fundraising for research and for the Society's other activities is
the responsibility of the Fundraising Department, actively
supported by branches and individual members throughout the
country. Currently they are managing to raise almost £5 million
each year, mainly from bequests and through special fundraising efforts.

Special interest groups

The YAPP&RS

Pronounced 'Yappers', this is the special interest group for
younger (ie those of working age) members of the Parkinson's
Disease Society (one in seven of all people diagnosed is under
the age of 40). The letters stand for Young Alert Parkinsonians,
Partners & Relatives. Since its beginnings in the late 1980s, its
membership (about 700 at the moment) and influence has
grown steadily and it is a very important source of support and
encouragement for its members. It is also a source of ideas and
energy for the Society as a whole and many of its members are
active in local branches.

The group produces its own lively quarterly magazine called

Yapmag and also organises a computerised bulletin board system (called *Shaking Hands*) which is available to everyone with Parkinson's and allows them to communicate with others in this country and around the world.

There are regional sub-groups of YAPP&RS in various parts of the country which arrange informal meetings. National meetings with invited speakers are arranged every one or two years and are usually held over a weekend. A very successful one, involving young Parkinsonians from all over Europe, was held at Peterborough in 1994.

Spring

Spring is another special interest group within the Parkinson's Disease Society. Its objective is to support and encourage medical research into Parkinson's and to keep its members informed about progress in research.

Glossary

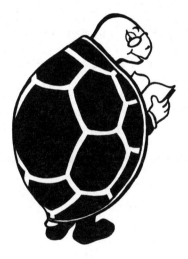

Terms in *italics* in these definitions refer to other terms in the glossary.

acetylcholine A chemical messenger found in the body that transmits messages between nerve cells or between nerve cells and muscles. These messages can affect the way muscles behave, or the amount of saliva produced. Because the actions of acetylcholine are called cholinergic actions, the drugs that block these actions are called *anticholinergic drugs*.

advocate A person who intercedes on behalf of another; someone who helps vulnerable or distressed people to make their voices heard.

agonists A term used for drugs which have a positive stimulating effect on particular cells in the body.

Alzheimer's disease The most common type of *dementia*.

anticholinergics A group of drugs used to treat Parkinson's, which work by reducing the amount of *acetylcholine* in the body, and so facilitate the function of dopamine cells. Drugs in this group are not now used as often as they were before the discovery of *L-dopa*.

anti-depressants Drugs given to treat *depression*.

apomorphine A *dopamine agonist* drug which is usually given by injection.

aromatherapy A *complementary therapy* involving treatment with *essential oils* – often involving massage, but the oils can also be inhaled or added to baths.

benign essential tremor Another name for *essential tremor*.

bradykinesia Slowness of movement.

carbohydrate A class of food which consists of starchy and sugary foods – examples include rice, bread, pasta, potatoes and dried beans.

cardiologist A doctor who specialises in the care and treatment of heart conditions.

care manager A person from a *Social Services department* (or sometimes from *Community Health Services*) who is given the task of putting together, monitoring and reviewing the plan of care agreed after a *community care assessment*.

carer In the broadest sense, a carer is anyone who provides help and support of any kind to a relative or friend. More specifically, a carer is a person who is regularly looking after someone who needs help with daily living (perhaps because of age or long-term illness) and who would not be able to live independently at home without this care and support.

choreiform movements Another name for *involuntary movements*.

clinical trials Closely-supervised scientific studies into treatments for diseases. A clinical trial may investigate a new treatment for a disease, or a different way of giving an existing treatment, or may compare a new treatment with the best treatment currently available.

communication aid Equipment which helps someone who has difficulty with speaking and/or writing to communicate more easily. Communication aids can vary from the very simple, such as alphabet boards or cards with messages already written on them, to the very complex, such as computers.

community care The provision of professional care and support to allow people who need help with daily living (perhaps because of age or long-term illness) to live as full and independent lives as possible (often in their own homes). The amount of care provided will depend on the needs and wishes of the person concerned (which must be taken into account) and on the resources which are available locally.

community care assessment The way in which professional staff from a *Social Services department* work out which *community care* services someone needs. The views of the person concerned and of their *carers* must be taken into account in making the assessment.

Community Health Councils or **CHCs** Each Health Authority has its own Community Health Council which is an independent voice on health care and is responsible for representing the interests of users of local health care services. CHC services range from providing information on what services are available locally to helping individuals who are unhappy with the service which they have received.

Community Health Services or **Community Health Trusts** The parts of the NHS which provide health care in people's own homes or in local clinics and health centres rather than in hospitals.

complementary therapies Non-medical treatments which may be used in addition to conventional medical treatments. Popular complementary therapies include *aromatherapy, homeopathy* and *osteopathy*. Some of these therapies are available through the NHS, but this is unusual, and depends on individual hospitals and GPs.

continuous care beds Beds, usually within hospitals but sometimes in *nursing homes*, which are funded by the NHS for people who need permanent medical care.

controlled release Special formulations of drugs that release the drug into the body slowly and steadily rather than all at once. They keep the amount of drug in the blood stream at a steadier level than the 'ordinary' version of the same drug.

corticobasal degeneration Also known as Steele-Richardson syndrome, progressive supra-nuclear palsy or striatonigral degeneration, this is one of the *Parkinson's Plus syndromes*.

counselling Counsellors are trained to listen carefully to what someone is saying about a particular problem or experience, and then to respond in a way which helps that person to explore and understand more clearly what they are thinking and feeling about that situation. Counselling therefore provides an opportunity for talking openly and fully about feelings without the worry of upsetting close friends or family members. It is always private and confidential.

CT scans An x-ray technique which helps doctors to diagnose disease. The x-rays are passed through the body from many different directions, and are then analysed by a computer to produce cross-sectional pictures of the body.

degeneration of nerve cells Death of nerve cells which cannot be explained by infection, blockage of blood vessels or failure of the immune system. Such degeneration is part of the ageing process but in conditions such as Parkinson's, it happens more rapidly than normal.

dementia A disorder in which the brain cells die more quickly than in normal ageing. The main symptoms are loss of memory and loss of the ability to do quite simple everyday tasks. The cells affected in dementia are **NOT** the cells that are affected in Parkinson's.

depression Feeling sad, hopeless, pessimistic, withdrawn and generally lacking interest in life. Most people feel depressed at some points in their lives, usually in reaction to a specific event such as a bereavement. Doctors become concerned when these feelings persist, especially when there was no obvious outside cause to trigger the feelings in the first place. The physical signs of depression include coping badly, losing weight and not responding well to medication: doctors may diagnose depression from these signs even in someone who claims not to feel depressed.

dietitian A health professional trained in nutrition who can provide advice and information on all aspects of diet and eating behaviour.

dopa-agonists Another name for *dopamine agonists*.

dopa-decarboxylase inhibitors Dopa-decarboxylase is a substance made in the body which converts *L-dopa* into *dopamine*. Dopa-decarboxylase inhibitors are drugs which stop this substance working until the L-dopa in the blood stream reaches the brain. This prevents the *side effects* which can occur if L-dopa is taken on its own.

dopamine A chemical messenger produced by cells in a part of the brain called the *substantia nigra*. Its function is to pass messages from the brain to other parts of the body, particularly to those parts involved in the coordination of movement. Dopamine is in short supply in people who have Parkinson's.

dopamine agonists A group of drugs used to treat Parkinson's. They work by stimulating the parts of the brain which use dopamine.

dopamine replacement therapy Treatment with drugs such as Madopar and Sinemet which contain *L-dopa*. When the L-dopa reaches the brain it is converted into *dopamine*, making up for the short supply of this chemical messenger in people with Parkinson's.

double-blind trials A type of *clinical trial* often used in testing the effectiveness of drugs and medicines. It ensures that neither the researcher nor the person taking part in the trial knows whether the drug being given in any individual case is the active medicine or a *placebo*. The aim of this type of trial is to make the research as objective as possible.

dribbling Another word for *drooling*.

driving assessment A test, which takes place at a specially staffed and equipped centre, of someone's ability and fitness to drive a car (with or without special adaptations).

drooling Having saliva overflowing from the mouth.

drug-induced Parkinson's Parkinson's-type symptoms caused by taking certain types of drugs, usually those used for severe psychiatric problems or dizziness. The symptoms wear off with time when the drugs are stopped. The term can also refer to the Parkinson's-like symptoms caused by drugs of abuse containing *MPTP*.

drug trials A name for *clinical trials* in which drugs are the treatments which are being tested.

dyskinesias Another name for *involuntary movements*.

dystonia An involuntary contraction of the muscles which causes the affected part of the body to go into a spasm (ie to twist or tighten). Such spasms can be painful and can produce abnormal movements, postures, or positions of the affected parts of the body.

encephalitis lethargica Encephalitis means inflammation of the brain and this particular type, which is caused by a virus, makes people very slow and tired (lethargic). It is rarely, if ever, seen now, but there was an epidemic of it after World War I. It often led to a particular type of Parkinson's called 'post-encephalitic Parkinson's'.

epidemiology A branch of medical research which tries to establish the frequency with which diseases occur. For example, it might be used to try to find out how many people in a population of 100,000 have Parkinson's, how many of these people are male and how many female, and how the people with Parkinson's are distributed among different age groups.

essential oils Aromatic (scented) oils extracted from the roots, flowers or leaves of plants by distillation. The complex chemicals in the oils can affect the nervous and circulatory systems of the body and so are considered to have therapeutic properties.

essential tremor A type of *tremor* which often runs in families and which is different from the tremor found in Parkinson's. Essential tremor is at its worst with the arms outstretched or when holding a cup of tea or writing, whereas the tremor of Parkinson's is usually most obvious when the arm is doing nothing and at rest.

familial tremor Another name for *essential tremor*.

foetal cell implants or **foetal implants** A much-publicised experimental technique involving implanting cells from aborted foetuses (unborn babies) into the brain of someone with Parkinson's in the hope of repairing the damage that the Parkinson's has caused. Although the technique has been quite successful in animals, its application to people with Parkinson's is still at the experimental stage.

free radicals Highly active chemical units which can be produced by the body or absorbed from outside sources (such as cigarette smoke or polluted air). They only last for very short periods of time, but have the potential to do damage to the body's cells during that time. The body has defence mechanisms against free radicals, but if it is unable to dispose of them fast enough, then cell damage results.

freezing The symptom, quite common in Parkinson's, which causes the person affected to stop suddenly while walking and to be unable to move forward for several seconds or minutes. It makes people feel that their feet are frozen to the ground.

genes The 'units' of heredity that determine our inherited characteristics, such as eye colour.

geriatrician A doctor who specialises in the care and treatment of elderly people.

glaucoma A disease affecting the eyes, usually found in older people. In glaucoma, the pressure of the fluid in the eye becomes so high that it causes damage, and the field of vision becomes progressively narrower and shallower. If left untreated, it can lead to blindness.

growth factors Natural substances produced in the body which help cells to grow in embryros and foetuses (unborn babies) and which also help adult cells to remain healthy. It is hoped that research into growth factors and the way they work may lead eventually to discovering ways of using these substances to help damaged cells in the brain and central nervous system to regenerate (repair themselves and grow again). Conditions such as Parkinson's which affect the brain and central nervous system are difficult to treat because cells in these parts of the body have very limited capacities for repair and regrowth. It might be possible in the future to use growth factors to make these cells behave more like cells in some other parts of the body (eg the skin) which already have the ability to regenerate.

home care worker Usually a person who provides help with personal care, such as getting washed and dressed, and with preparing meals. Home care workers are normally provided by *Social Services departments*, and there is usually a charge for their services.

home help Usually a person who provides help with shopping, cleaning and similar household tasks but who does not usually provide personal care. Home helps are normally provided by *Social Services departments*, and there is usually a charge for their services.

homeopathy A *complementary therapy* based on the principle that 'like can be cured by like' (the word homeopathy comes from two Greek words that mean 'similar' and 'suffering'). The remedies used (which are completely safe) contain very dilute amounts of a substance which in larger quantities would produce similar symptoms to the illness being treated. Although there is as yet no scientific explanation for why homeopathy works, it is available through the NHS, although the provision is limited.

idiopathic A word used before the name of an illness or medical condition which means that its cause is not known.

impotence Failure of erection of the penis.

inhibitors A term used for drugs which have a blocking effect on particular cells or chemical reactions in the body.

involuntary movements Movements, other than *tremor*, which are not willed or intended by the person affected. They tend to occur in people who have had Parkinson's for many years and to be related, often in complex and variable ways, to the timing of medication.

L-dopa A substance one step removed from *dopamine*. It is not possible for dopamine to pass from the blood stream to the brain, so the problem is solved by giving drugs containing L-dopa. The L-dopa can reach the brain from the blood stream, and when it gets there it is converted into dopamine.

levodopa Another name for *L-dopa*.

Lewy body A microscopic structure seen in the brains of people with Parkinson's.

local ethics committee A group of doctors, researchers and lay people who check the plans of medical researchers to make sure that the interests of people who take part in research projects are protected. Each Health Authority has its own local ethics committee.

mask face Another name for *poker face*.

micrographia The technical name for small handwriting. It comes from two Greek words, 'mikros' meaning little and 'graphein' meaning to write.

mitochondria A part of each cell in the body. It is the 'power pack' of the cell and if it is damaged the cell dies.

monoamine oxidase B A naturally-occurring chemical found in the body which causes the breakdown of *dopamine*.

MPTP A poisonous chemical contained in some drugs of abuse used by young American drug addicts in the early 1980s. It produced an illness with symptoms very similar to those found in Parkinson's.

multi-disciplinary assessment An assessment, involving medical, nursing, therapy and Social Services personnel, of the medical and social care/support someone needs. It is called multi-disciplinary simply because professionals from several different disciplines or specialities are involved!

multiple system atrophy Also known as Shy-Drager syndrome, this is one of the *Parkinson's Plus syndromes*.

music therapy The use, by trained professionals, of music as treatment for certain physical and mental illnesses. The music can be used to improve mobility and speech and to enable people to relax or to express feelings and ideas. Music therapists often work with *physical therapists*.

neurological conditions Conditions affecting the body's nervous system (ie the brain and associated nerves).

neurologist A doctor who specialises in the diagnosis, care and treatment of diseases of the nervous system (ie the brain and associated nerves).

nursing homes *Residential homes* which offer continuous 24-hour nursing care.

occupational therapists Trained professionals who use specific, selected tasks and activities to enable people who have difficulty with control and coordination of movement to attain maximum function and independence. They also assess people's homes and places of work and suggest ways of making them safer and more manageable. Occupational therapists advise on special aids and gadgets to help with the practical problems of daily living, and on leisure activities to help improve the quality of daily life.

on/off phenomenon This phenomenon is characteristic of some people with long-standing Parkinson's. It can cause them to change from being 'on' and able to move, to being 'off' and virtually immobile, all within a very brief period of time – minutes or even seconds.

osteopathy *A complementary therapy* involving manipulation of the bones and muscles. It is most commonly used for back pain, joint pain and stiffness, and similar conditions.

oxygen free radicals *Free radicals* of oxygen.

pallidotomy An operation on the pallidum, which is a part of the brain concerned with movement. This type of *stereotactic surgery* was originally developed in the 1950s but fell out of favour during the next 30 years. It is now is attracting renewed interest and research.

Parkinson's Plus syndromes Rare conditions whose early symptoms look like Parkinson's but later develop in rather different ways.

pavement vehicle A motorised wheelchair or scooter suitable for use outdoors.

Penject A type of small portable syringe which looks rather like a pen (hence the name), made by Hypoguard Ltd and used for apomorphine injections. The syringe delivers a pre-measured dose when a button on it is pressed.

PET scans The only type of scan that can 'show' Parkinson's. As yet it is only available in some research centres.

physical therapies A group of therapies which includes *occupational therapy, physiotherapy* and *speech and language therapy.*

physiotherapy Physical treatments (including exercises) which are used to prevent or reduce stiffness in joints and to restore muscle strength.

placebo The name given in *double-blind trials* to the non-active substance with which an active drug is being compared. It is a 'dummy' version of the drug, identical in appearance to the drug being tested.

poker face Lack of the facial expressions that indicate emotions, for example frowning and smiling.

progressive supra-nuclear palsy Also known as Steele-Richardson syndrome, striatonigral degeneration or corticobasal degeneration, this is one of the *Parkinson's Plus syndromes.*

protein A class of food that is necessary for the growth and repair of the body's tissues – examples include fish, meat, eggs and milk.

residential homes Accommodation for people who are no longer able or who no longer wish to manage everyday domestic tasks (such as cooking, shopping, housework and so on) or to maintain an independent home of their own, but who do not need nursing care.

respite care Any facility or resource which allows those who care for sick, frail, elderly or disabled relatives or friends to have a break from their caring tasks. Respite care may be provided in residential or nursing homes, in the person's own home, or with another family.

resting tremor A name sometimes used for the type of *tremor* found in Parkinson's.

restless leg syndrome Legs that regularly burn, prickle or ache, especially in bed at night. The cause is not known.

rigidity The name given to the special type of stiffness which is one of the main symptoms of Parkinson's. The muscles tend to pull against each other instead of working smoothly together.

season ticket Shorthand name for a prepayment certificate for NHS prescriptions.

self-referral Going direct to a therapist for treatment rather than through a GP or other health professional.

sheltered housing Accommodation which is purpose-built for people who need a certain amount of supervision because of old age or disability, but who wish to maintain a home of their own. The amount of supervision available can vary from a warden on site who can be contacted in an emergency to high-dependency units where there is still a degree of privacy and independence, but where higher staffing levels allow assistance with meals and personal care.

Shy-Drager syndrome Also known as multiple system atrophy, this is one of the *Parkinson's Plus syndromes*.

side effects Almost all drugs affect the body in ways beyond their intended therapeutic actions. These unwanted 'extra' effects are called side effects. Side effects vary in their severity from person to person, and often disappear when the body becomes used to a particular drug.

sleeping sickness In this book, another name for *encephalitis lethargica*.

senile tremor Another name for *essential tremor*.

Social Services departments The departments of local authorities responsible for non-medical welfare care for children and adults who need such help.

speech and language therapists Trained professionals who help with problems concerning speech, communication or swallowing.

Steele-Richardson syndrome Also known as progressive supra-nuclear palsy, striatonigral degeneration or corticobasal degeneration, this is one of the *Parkinson's Plus syndromes*.

stereotactic or **stereotaxic surgery** Type of brain surgery which involves inserting delicate instruments through a specially created small hole in the skull, and then using these instruments to operate on deep structures in the brain which are concerned with the control of movement. The forms of sterotactic surgery which are very occasionally used in Parkinson's are *pallidotomy* and *thalamotomy*.

striatonigral degeneration Also known as Steele-Richardson syndrome, progressive supra-nuclear palsy or corticobasal degeneration, this is one of the *Parkinson's Plus syndromes*.

subcutaneous Under the skin.

substantia nigra So-called because of its dark colour (the name literally means 'black substance'), this part of the brain coordinates movement and contains cells that make *dopamine*. It is cells from the substantia nigra which are lost or damaged in Parkinson's.

syringe driver A small, battery driven pump which can deliver a continuous dose of medication through a flexible line (fine tube) which ends in a needle which is inserted under the skin. It allows people with serious *on/off* Parkinson's to receive a continuous infusion of *apomorphine* and to top this up with occasional booster doses as necessary.

thalamus A part of the brain (located near the *substantia nigra*) which is responsible for relaying information from the sense organs about what is going on in the body to the various parts of the brain.

thalamotomy A type of *stereotactic surgery* performed on the *thalamus*. It was used quite extensively in the past (before the advent of *L-dopa* and *dopamine replacement therapy*) in the treatment of one-sided *tremor*, but is rarely used nowadays.

tissue bank A collection of body tissues which can be used for research purposes. People interested in supporting a tissue bank sign an agreement during their lifetime; the tissue is then donated to the bank after their death. Tissue banks are very important research resources, and the Parkinson's Disease Society has its own Brain Tissue Bank.

tremor Involuntary shaking, trembling or quivering movements of the muscles. It is caused by the muscles alternately contracting and relaxing at a rapid rate.

wearing off phenomenon In this phenomenon, which is characteristic of some people with long-standing Parkinson's, the effectiveness of the drug treatment is substantially reduced so that it 'wears off' some time before the next dose is due.

yo-yoing Another name for the *on/off phenomenon*.

Appendix 1

Useful addresses

Age Concern England
Astral House
1268 London Road
London SW16 4ER
Tel: 0181 679 8000

Age Concern Scotland
54A Fountainbridge
Edinburgh EH3 9PT
Tel: 0131 228 5656

AREMCO Swivel cushions
Grove House
Lenham
Kent ME17 2PX
Tel: 01622 858502

Association of Crossroads Care
  Attendant Schemes
10 Regent Place
Rugby
Warks CV21 2PN
Tel: 01788 573653

Association of Professional
  Music Therapists
38 Pierce Lane
Fulbourn
Cambs CB1 5DL
Tel: 01223 880377

Banstead Mobility Centre
Damson Way
Orchard Hill
Queen Mary's Avenue
Carshalton
Surrey SM5 4NR
Tel: 0181 770 1151

Benefits Agency
Chief Executive's Office
Room 4C06
Quarry House
Quarry Hill
Leeds LS2 7UA

Brain Tissue Bank
Institute of Neurology
1 Wakefield Street
London WC1N 1PJ
Tel: 0171 837 8370

British Complementary
    Medicine Association
St Charles Hospital
Exmoor Street
London W10 6DZ
Tel: 0181 964 1205

British Society of Dentistry for
    the Handicapped
c/o Mrs Sue Greening
Dental Department
Town Centre Clinic
Caradoc Road
Cwmbran
Gwent NP44 1XG
Tel: 01633 838356

British Sports Association for
    the Disabled
Mary Glen Haig Suite
Solecast House
13–27 Brunswick Place
London N1 6DX
Tel: 0171 490 1919

Canon Communicators
Canon UK Ltd
Canon House
Manor Road
Wallington
Surrey SM6 0AJ
Tel: 0181 773 3173

Carers National Association
20/25 Glasshouse Yard
London EC1A 4JS
Tel: 0171 490 8818
Helpline: Tel: 0171 490 8898

Chester-Care
Sidings Road
Low Moor Estate
Kirkby-in-Ashfield
Notts NG17 7JZ
Tel: 01623 757955

Chivers Large Print Books
Chivers Press Ltd
Windsor Bridge Road
Bath BA2 3AX
Tel: 01225 335336

Computability Centre
PO Box 94
Warwick CV34 5WS
Tel: 01926 312847
Freephone Advice Line: 0800
    269545

Continence Foundation
2 Doughty Street
London WC1N 2PH
Tel: 0171 404 6875

Continence Advisory Service
    Helpline
Tel: 0191 213 0050 (2pm – 7pm
    weekdays)

Counsel and Care
Lower Ground Floor
Twyman House
16 Bonny Street
London NW1 9PG
Tel: 0171 485 1566 (10.30am –
   4.00pm)

Crossroads Scotland Care
   Attendant Schemes
24 George Square
Glasgow G2 1EG
Tel: 0141 226 3793

DIAL UK
St Catherine's Hospital
Tickhill Road
Balby
Doncaster DN4 8QN
Tel: 01302 310123

Disabled Living Centres
   Council
286 Camden Road
London N7 0BT
Tel: 0171 700 1707

Disabled Living Foundation
380/384 Harrow Road
London W9 2HU
Tel: 0171 289 6111

DVLA
(Driver and Vehicle Licensing
   Agency)
Drivers' Medical Unit
Longview Road
Morriston
Swansea SA99 1TU
Tel: 01792 783686

Gardening for the Disabled
   Trust
c/o F Seton
The Freight
Cranbrook
Kent TN17 3PG
Tel: 01580 712196

General Council and Register
   of Osteopaths
56 London Street
Reading
Berkshire RG1 4SQ
Tel: 01734 576585

Health Education Authority
Hamilton House
Mabledon Place
London WC1H 9TX
Tel: 0171 383 3833

Holiday Care Service
2 Old Bank Chambers
Station Road
Horley
Surrey RH6 9HW
Tel: 01293 774535

Horticultural Therapy
Goulds Ground
Vallis Way
Frome
Somerset BA11 3DW
Tel: 01373 464782

Institute for Complementary
   Medicine
PO Box 194
London SE16 1AA
Tel: 0171 237 5165

Keep Able Ltd
For a mail order catalogue,
write to:
Keep Able Ltd
FREEPOST
Wellingborough
Northants NN8 6BR
Shops at:
2 Capital Interchange Way
Brentford
Middlesex TW8 0EX
Tel: 0181 742 2181
and
Sterling Park
Pedmore Road
Brierley Hill
West Midlands DY5 1TA
Tel: 01384 484544
and
Fleming Close
Park Farm
Wellingborough
Northants NN8 6UF
Tel: 01933 679426

Leonard Cheshire Foundation
26/29 Maunsel Street
London SW1P 2QW
Tel: 0171 828 1822

Lightwriters
Toby Churchill Ltd
20 Panton Street
Cambridge CB1 1HP
Tel: 01223 316117

Mobility Assessment Centres
Details about your nearest
centre can be obtained from:
Mobility Advice & Vehicle
    Information Service (MAVIS)
Department of Transport
TRL
Crowthorne
Berks RG11 6AU
Tel: 01344 770456
or
Disabled Drivers' Motor Club
Cottingham Way
Thrapston
Northants NN14 4PL
Tel: 01832 734724

Motability
Gate House
Westgate
Harlow
Essex CM20 1HR
Tel: 01279 635666

National Listening Library
12 Lant Street
London SE1 1BR
Tel: 0171 407 9417

Open University (OU)
General enquiries:
Central Enquiry Office
PO Box 200
Milton Keynes MK7 6YZ
Tel: 01908 653231

Open University (*contd.*)
For special advice:
Adviser on the Education of
    Disabled Students
Regional Academic Services
Walton Hall
Milton Keynes MK7 6AA
Tel: 01908 653442

Parkinson's Disease Society
    (PDS)
National Office
22 Upper Woburn Place
London WC1H 0RA
Tel: 0171 383 3513
Helpline: 0171 388 5798

Parkinson's Disease Society
    Brain Tissue Bank
Institute of Neurology
1 Wakefield Street
London WC1N 1PJ
Tel: 0171 837 8370

RADAR
(Royal Association for
    Disability and Rehabilitation)
12 City Forum
250 City Road
London EC1V 8AF
Tel: 0171 250 3222

Rail Unit for Disabled
    Passengers Switchboard
Tel: 0171 928 5151

Relate
Herbert Gray College
Little Church Street
Rugby
Warwickshire CV21 3AP
Tel: 01788 573241/560811

Research Council for
    Complementary Medicine
60 Great Ormond Street
London WC1N 3JF
Tel: 0171 833 8897

Shirley Price Aromatherapy
    Ltd
Essentia House
Upper Bond Street
Hinkley
Leics LE10 1RS
Tel: 01455 615466

Silky sheets supplier
Greens
80/84 Seven Sisters Road
Holloway
London N7 6AE
Tel: 0171 607 6310

SPOD
(Association to aid the Sexual
    and Personal Relationships
    of People with a Disability)
286 Camden Road
London N7 0BJ
Tel: 0171 607 8851

Swivel car seats suppliers
ELAP Engineering Limited
Fort Street
Accrington
Lancs BB5 1QG
Tel: 01254 871599
Addresses of other suppliers
available from Disabled
Living Centres

Talking Newspapers
    Association UK
National Recording Centre
Heathfield
East Sussex TN21 8DB
Tel: 01435 866102

Technabed
Llewellyn Community Care
1 Regent Road
City
Liverpool L3 7BX
Tel: 0151 236 5311

Telecottage Association
Freephone: 0800 616 008

Tripscope
65 Esmond Road
London W4 1JE
Tel: 0181 994 9294

Ulverscroft Large Print Books
F A Thorpe Publishing Ltd
Anstey
Leicestershire LE7 7FU
Tel: 01533 364325

University of the Third Age
1 Stockwell Green
London SW9 9JF
Tel: 0171 737 2541

Walsall Residential Home for
    People with Parkinson's
Mali Jenkins House
The Crescent
Walsall
West Midlands WS1 2BX
Enquiries and applications to:
John White
The Greytree Trust
Greytree Lodge
Second Avenue
Ross-on-Wye
Herefordshire HR9 7HT
Tel: 01989 562630

Winged Fellowship Trust
Angel House
20/32 Pentonville Road
London N1 9XD
Tel 0171 833 2594

Writers' Own Publications
Eileen M Pickering (Editor)
121 Highbury Grove
Clapham
Bedford MK41 6DU
Tel: 01234 65982

Yoga for Health Foundation
Ickwell Bury
Biggleswade
Beds SG18 9EF
Tel: 01767 27271

Appendix 2

Useful publications

At the time of writing, all the publications listed here were available. Where a title has been mentioned in this book, it is marked with an asterisk (*).

We have indicated the titles that are available free of charge; for all other items we suggest that you check current prices with your local bookshop or with the publishers. Your local library may have copies of some of the books mentioned, either for loan or as reference copies.

Parkinson's Disease Society publications

Free booklets

Single copies of the following booklets are available free from the Parkinson's Disease Society (address in Appendix 1) on receipt of a large (at least 16 × 23 cm or 9 × 7 in) stamped addressed envelope.

Coping with Parkinson's (introductory booklet)

* The Drug Treatment of Parkinson's Disease: notes for patients and their families

Parkinson's Disease: a booklet for patients and their families, by Dr R.B. Godwin-Austen

Parkinson's Disease Day to Day

* Parkinson's Disease and Sex

* Speech Therapy and your Speech/Language Therapist

Publications for which there is a charge
Please check with the Parkinson's Disease Society (address in Appendix 1) for current prices.

* Bowls for the Parkinsonian, by Alex Flinder (Mali Jenkins essay prize-winner)

* Face to Face (video cassette and booklet), by Iona Lister

* Information Pack for Nurses

* Introducing a self administration of drugs programme to improve the quality of life for clients with Parkinson's Disease whilst in hospital, by Bernadette Porter (Mali Jenkins essay prize-winner)

* Living with Parkinson's Disease, by Sue Franklyn, Alison Perry and Alison Beattie

  Physiotherapy exercise (audiocassette tape)

  Relaxation (audiocassette tape)

  Speech exercises (audiocassette tape)

Books about Parkinson's

Parkinson's Disease: a guide for the patient and his family, by R.C. Duvoisin, published by Raven Press (USA)

Parkinson's Disease, by Dr Harvey Sagar, published by Optima

Books by and about people with Parkinson's

Parkinson's: a patient's view, by Sidney Dorros, published by Seven Locks Press Inc (USA)

Living Well with Parkinson's, by G. Wotton Attwood with L. Green Hunnewell, published by John Wiley & Sons Ltd.

Ray of Hope, by Andrew Lees and Ray Kennedy, published by Pelham Books

Clothing and useful equipment

* Advice Notes for People with Parkinson's Disease (resource paper), published jointly by the Disabled Living Foundation and the Parkinson's Disease Society (obtainable from the Parkinson's Disease Society)

* Clothing for People with Parkinson's Disease, published by Disability Scotland (obtainable free of charge from the Parkinson's Disease Society)

Equipment for an Easier Life, published by RICA (Research Institute for Consumer Affairs), 2 Marylebone Road, London NW1 4DF (single copies available free of charge on receipt of an A5 SAE)

* Keep Able Mail Order Catalogue, obtainable free of charge from Keep Able Ltd at the address given in Appendix 1

The Special Collection (a mail order catalogue of fashion clothing selected for people with dressing difficulties), obtainable free of charge from J.D. Williams, Freepost, PO Box 123, Manchester M99 1BN (Tel: 0161 237 1200)

Publications about leisure activities

* National Trust Handbook (a new edition is published each year – it is available free to members and is also on sale in bookshops)

* National Gardens Scheme Handbook (a new edition is published each year – it is available free to members and is also on sale in bookshops and newsagents)

* Places That Care, by M.B. Yarrow, published by Mediair Marketing Services, 72 High St, Poole, Dorset BH15 1DA (Tel: 01202 671545)

* Historic Houses, Castles and Gardens, published by British Leisure Publications, Windsor Court, East Grinstead, West Sussex RH19 1XA (Tel: 01342 326972)

* Cook It Yourself: Cooking with a Physical Disability, by M. Berriedale-Johnson and A. Davies, published by Cedar

* Grow It Yourself: Gardening with a Physical Disability, by R. Llewellyn and A. Davies, published by Cedar

Publications about mobility

Door to Door, published by the Department of Transport (available free of charge from the Mobility Advice and Vehicle Information Service – MAVIS – at the address in Appendix 1)

RADAR factsheets
Copies of the following factsheets are available from RADAR (address

in Appendix 1). The cost is 75p each or three for £2.00 (postage included).

1. Motoring with a wheelchair
2. Exemption from Vehicle Excise Duty (VED)
3. Relief from VAT and Car Tax
4. Driving licences
5. Assessment Centres and driving instruction
* 6. Insurance
7. Motoring accessories
* 8. Cash help for mobility needs
9. Discounts and concessions available to disabled people on the purchase of cars and other related items
10. Car control manufacturers, suppliers and fitters

Publications for carers

Caring at Home, by Nancy Kohner, commissioned by the King's Fund Centre Carers Unit and published by the National Extension College, 18 Brooklands Avenue, Cambridge CB2 2HN

* Taking a Break, published by the King's Fund Carers Unit (single copy free to carers available from Taking a Break, Newcastle-upon-Tyne X, NE85 2AQ)

* What to look for in a Private or Voluntary Registered Home (Factsheet Number 5), published by Counsel and Care, Lower Ground Floor, Twyman House, 16 Bonny Street, London NW1 9PG (Tel: 0171 485 1566)

Taking Time for Me: How Caregivers Can Deal Effectively with Stress, by K.L. Karr, published by Prometheus Books

* Coping with Dementia: a Handbook for Carers, published by Health Education Board Scotland, Woodburn House, Canaan Lane, Edinburgh EH10 4SG (Tel: 0131 447 8044) (Single copies are available free from local Health Boards in Scotland. People from outside Scotland can purchase copies - please telephone first to check the cost)

Caring for the Person with Dementia, by Bob Woods and Chris Lay, published by the Alzheimer's Disease Society, 10 Greencoat Place, London SW1P 1PH (Tel: 0171 306 0606) (There is a charge for this publication, but the Society also publishes a number of useful free leaflets, which are available directly from them or from their local branches)

* Age Concern Factsheet Number 22: Legal Arrangements for Managing Financial Affairs (separate versions for England and Wales and for Scotland available from the relevant Age Concern offices at the addresses in Appendix 1)

Other publications

* BT Guide for Elderly or Disabled People (available free on request by calling Freefone 0800 800 150)

* Patient's Charter, published by the Department of Health (contact your local Health Authority for a free copy)

* Traveller's Guide to Health, published by the Department of Health (single copies available free on request by calling Freefone 0800 555 777)

Reference books for consultation at your local library

* Charities Digest, published by the Family Welfare Association (updated every year)

* A Guide to Grants for Individuals in Need, published by the Directory of Social Change (updated every other year)

* Which? the monthly magazine of the Consumers' Association (the article on *Choosing a Care Home appears on pages 46-47 of the August 1994 issue)

Index

221

PRIORITY ORDER FORM

Cut out or photocopy this form and send it (post free in the UK) to:

Class Publishing Customer Service
FREEPOST (no stamp needed)
LONDON W6 7BR

Tel: 01752 695745

Fax: 01752 695668

Please send me urgently
(tick boxes below)

**Post included
price per copy
(UK only)**

☐ **Parkinson's at your fingertips**
(ISBN: 1 872362 47 8) £14.95

☐ **Epilepsy at your fingertips**
(ISBN: 1 872362 51 6) £14.95

☐ **Asthma at your fingertips**
(ISBN: 1 872362 06 0) £14.95

☐ **Allergies at your fingertips**
(ISBN: 1 872362 52 4) £14.95

☐ **High blood pressure at your fingertips**
(ISBN: 1 872362 48 6) £14.95

☐ **Diabetes at your fingertips**
(ISBN: 1 872362 49 4) £14.95

☐ **Cancer information at your fingertips**
(ISBN: 1 872362 09 5) £11.95

TOTAL: _____

Easy ways to pay
Cheque: I enclose a cheque payable to Class Publishing for £_____
Credit card: please debit my Access ☐ Visa ☐ Amex ☐ Switch ☐

Number: _____ Expiry date: _____

Name: _____

Address: _____

_____

Town: _____ County: _____ Postcode: _____

My telephone number (in case of queries): _____

Class Publishing's guarantee: remember that if, for any reason, you are not satisfied with these books, we will refund all your money, without any questions asked. Prices and VAT rates may be altered for reasons beyond our control.

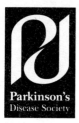

Parkinson's
Disease Society

Parkinson's Disease Society of the United Kingdom

The Society's mission is: The conquest of Parkinson's disease and the alleviation of the suffering and distress it causes, through effective research, welfare, education and communication.

We aim:
- to help patients and their relatives with the problems arising from Parkinson's disease
- to collect and disseminate information on Parkinson's disease
- to encourage and provide funds for research into Parkinson's disease.

For help and advice about Parkinson's disease, please contact the Society at the address given below. An information pack which includes a list of our local branches can be obtained from the Society by completing this form.

☐ Please send me an information pack about the Parkinson's Disease Society.

☐ Please send me a membership form.

Individual subscription (including quarterly newsletter)   £3.00.

Subscription rate for professionals, etc on request.

The Parkinson's Disease Society always need donations and practical help. Some ways in which you can help are listed below.

☐ I would like to be a volunteer.

☐ Please may I have a covenant form.

☐ Please send me information about legacies.

☐ I enclose a donation for £ _____.

Cheques/postal orders should be made payable to the Parkinson's Disease Society.

An A5 SAE with stamps to the value of 43p would be appreciated.

Name _____

Address _____

_____

Postcode _____ Telephone _____

Please return this form to: The Parkinson's Disease Society, 22 Upper Woburn Place, London WC1H 0RA. Telephone: 0171 383 3513. Helpline: 0171 388 5798 (Mondays–Fridays 10.00–4.00) Fax: 0171 383 5754.